The ECT Handbook

The Second Report of the Royal College of Psychiatrists' Special Committee on ECT

The ECT Handbook

The Second Report of the Royal College of
Psychiatrists' Special Committee on ECT

Edited by C. P. Freeman

Council Report CR39
January 1995

Royal College of Psychiatrists
London

Due for renewal: January 2000

© 1995 Royal College of Psychiatrists

First printed 1995
Reprinted 1996, 1998

Approved by the Council of the Royal College of Psychiatrists, January 1995.

British Library Cataloguing-in-Publication Data
ECT. – 1995: Second Report of the Royal
College of Psychiatrists' Special
Committee on ECT. – (Council Report: CR39)
    I. Freeman, Chris II. Series
    616.89122

ISBN 0 902241 83 4

College Reports

Reports produced by the Royal College of Psychiatrists and made available for general distribution fall into two categories: Council Reports and Occasional Papers. Council Reports have been approved by a meeting of Council and constitute official College policy. They are given blue covers, and are numbered CR1, CR2, etc. Occasional Papers have not been approved by Council, and do not constitute College policy. They are produced by departments or Sections of the College, and their distribution has been authorised by the College Officers with the aim of providing information or provoking discussion. They are numbered OP1, OP2, etc.

    Reports are available from the Publications Department at the Royal College of Psychiatrists, 17 Belgrave Square, London SW1X 8PG (tel. 0171 235 2351, fax 0171 245 1231).

Printed in Great Britain by Henry Ling Ltd., at the Dorset Press, Dorchester

Contents

Introduction   vi

Part I. Clinical guidelines

1   ECT and depressive disorders. *A. Scott*   3
2   ECT in mania. *J. Pippard*   6
3   ECT in schizophrenia. *T. Lock*   8
4   ECT as a specific treatment for neuropsychiatric conditions.   11
    T. Lock & R. McClelland
5   ECT in the elderly patient. *S. M. Benbow*   17
6   ECT in those under 18 years old. *C. P. Freeman*   18
7   ECT and obstetrics. *T. Lock*   22
8   ECT in learning disability psychiatry. *R. McClelland*   24
9   Safe ECT practice in physically ill patients. *S. M. Benbow*   26
10   ECT, violence and other offending behaviour. *P. Taylor*   30
11   Non-convulsive electric shock treatment. *T. Lock*   31
12   ECT and other conditions. *T. Lock & R. McClelland*   33

Part II. Administration of ECT

13   The ECT suite. *C. P. Freeman & J. Lambourn*   37
14   Equipment for the ECT suite. *G. Fergusson*   39
15   Anaesthesia for ECT. *K. H. Simpson*   42
16   ECT and drugs. *S. Curran & C. P. Freeman*   49
17   Prescribing. *C. P. Freeman*   58
18   Electrode placement: unilateral versus bilateral. *C. P. Freeman*   60
19   Monitoring seizure activity. *A. Scott & T. Lock*   62
20   Adverse effects of ECT. *S. M. Benbow*   67
21   Continuation ECT (maintenance ECT). *A. Scott*   71
22   Stimulus dosing. *T. Lock*   72
23   Electrical and neurophysiological principles. *T. Lock*   88
24   Training and supervision. *A. Scott*   94

Part III. The law and consent

25   ECT, the law and consent to treatment. *J. Pippard & P. Taylor*   97

Appendices

I   A factsheet for you and your family   103
II   Additional information for out-patients receiving ECT   106
III   The ECT treatment record form. *T. Lock*   107
IV   Consent form   113
V   Nursing guidelines for ECT. *S. M. Halsall, T. Lock & A. Atkinson*   114
VI   Review of ECT machines. *T. Lock*   122

Index   149

Introduction

This set of guidelines replaces *The Practical Administration of Electroconvulsive Therapy* (London: Royal College of Psychiatrists, 1989). It is essentially a practical set of guidelines for psychiatrists who will be prescribing or administering ECT. It is not a comprehensive textbook, but we have included brief reviews on the main clinical indications for ECT.

In order to keep these guidelines up-to-date, we will produce appendices covering new developments such as the introduction of new ECT machines and the development of new ECT techniques.

The Royal College of Psychiatrists will continue to run training courses on ECT on a regular basis. A separate teaching video is available from the Royal College. This covers some of the same material as these guidelines, but is intended specifically for consultant psychiatrists who are responsible for the running of an ECT department.

My thanks go to all the contributors who have worked so hard to produce these guidelines and particularly to the core members of the Special Committee on ECT:

Dr Susan Benbow
Dr Toni Lock
Professor Roy McClelland
Dr John Pippard
Dr Allan Scott

and more recently:

Dr Grace Fergusson
Dr Carol Robertson

My special thanks to Debbie Parish who supported the Committee through its many meetings, dealt with our many drafts and our idiosyncrasies, and kept us admirably to task.

Dr C. P. Freeman
Chairman
Special Committee on ECT
October 1994

Part I. Clinical guidelines

1. ECT and depressive disorders

A. Scott

The College "Memorandum on the use of electroconvulsive therapy" (1977) concluded that there was "substantial and incontrovertible evidence that the ECT procedure is an effective treatment in severe depressive illness". In the UK alone, there have been five further careful, double-blind, clinical comparisons of bilateral real and simulated ECT, all demonstrating the clear therapeutic benefit of real ECT as compared with the whole procedure minus the stimulus and seizure (Freeman *et al*, 1978; Johnstone *et al*, 1980; West, 1981; Brandon *et al*, 1984; Gregory *et al*, 1985).

Depressive illness is probably best viewed as a syndrome rather than a single pathological entity, because it can occur in the course of unipolar and bipolar affective disorders, post-partum, after adverse life events, and so on. The best predictor of the likelihood of a good response to ECT in a depressive syndrome is the number of the typical symptoms and signs of depressive illness (Abrams, 1992). A subsequent analysis of the combined data from the Leicester and Northwick Park trials found that ECT, as opposed to simulated ECT, was of specific value in the treatment of patients who displayed psychomotor retardation and/or depressive delusions or hallucinations (Buchan *et al*, 1992). There are no biological measures that have been shown to be superior to clinical criteria in the selection of depressed patients who will respond well to ECT (Scott, 1989).

There have been only a few direct comparisons of the efficacy of antidepressant drug treatment and ECT, and all have methodological shortcomings (Abrams, 1992). The large random-allocation studies by Greenblatt *et al* (1964) and the Medical Research Council (1965) found that treatment outcome after ECT was superior to that after imipramine, phenelzine or placebo. Unfortunately, the first study included patients with a variety of diagnoses and the second study used doses of antidepressant drugs that would now be considered potentially sub-therapeutic. The small random allocation study by Gangadhar *et al* (1982) was important because bilateral ECT plus placebo tablets were compared with sham ECT and imipramine; the improvement in depression ratings was significantly greater in patients treated by ECT after six treatments. This study was the best evidence to date that ECT works more quickly than antidepressant drug treatment, but can be criticised because the dose of imipramine during the first week of treatment was only 75 mg daily. This is clearly a topic that merits further research because one of the justifications for the use of ECT is that it works more quickly than antidepressant drug treatment.

Clinical experience suggested that depressed patients who had not responded to antidepressant drug treatment could recover if treated subsequently by ECT. This clinical impression has been confirmed by a well-conducted study by Prudic *et al* (1990), but the recovery rate is less than that seen in depressed patients who have not already had a trial of drug treatment before ECT.

How the speed of action of ECT is modified by the prescribing habits of psychiatrists has received little research interest, although the available evidence was recently reviewed (Scott & Whalley, 1993). Pippard & Ellam (1981) noted that a small minority of psychiatrists prescribed a fixed course of treatment without clinical review between treatments, presumably reflecting the clinical impression that there is a delay in the onset of any antidepressant effect. There is no empirical support for this clinical impression, and patients who recover with a course of ECT can show marked improvement after only a few treatments (Rodger *et al*, 1994). A set number of treatments should not be prescribed.

There is no research evidence that can give guidance on when ECT should be discontinued if no response at all has occurred. To some extent this will depend on the severity and/or chronicity of the depressive disorder. The range lies between 6 and 12 consecutive treatments. The previous guidelines suggested a maximum of eight *properly administered* treatments in the absence of any clinical improvement, although the American Psychiatric Association (1990) has advised that the indication for more ECT be re-assessed after 6–10 treatments. Occasionally, in patients with severe treatment-resistant depression, longer courses of ECT may be justified. Whenever a patient with the typical features of depressive illness shows little or no improvement after several ECT treatments, it is essential to review the factors that influence the speed of response to ECT, for example, electrode placement, stimulus dosing and concomitant drug treatment (see checklists).

ECT is usually given twice weekly in the UK, but three times a week in the US. The only published comparison of twice and thrice weekly bilateral ECT used the sine-wave stimulation in depressed patients with melancholia and found that twice-weekly ECT worked just as quickly as treatment three times a week (Gangadhar *et al*, 1993); whether this finding can be generalised to modern brief-pulse ECT is not known. It may be that, for most depressed patients, twice-weekly bilateral ECT is sufficient and appropriate. The earlier studies that compared different frequencies of unilateral ECT have methodological shortcomings, but neither four times weekly (Strömgren, 1975) nor thrice-weekly (McAllister *et al*, 1987) have been shown to induce improvement more quickly than twice-weekly treatment. In the management of severely ill patients, where ECT may be life-saving, two different strategies have been suggested to increase the rate of improvement. The first is to increase the frequency of treatment, even up to daily sessions, and the second strategy is to induce two seizures during the one anaesthetisation. These strategies have not been adequately assessed and should be regarded as experimental.

The debate about whether or not ECT causes permanent intellectual impairment or brain damage was recently reviewed (Abrams, 1992). Prospective magnetic resonance imaging in depressed patients treated by ECT has found no evidence of cortical atrophy or ventricular enlargement (Coffey *et al*, 1991) and no changes suggestive of parenchymal disorder of the cerebral hemispheres (Scott *et al*, 1991).

Continuation antidepressant drug treatment is essential after successful ECT because nearly half of the depressed patients who recover with ECT will relapse within 12 weeks without drug treatment (Barton *et al*, 1973). Patients who received ECT because they had already failed to respond to antidepressant drug treatment are also more likely to relapse in the months after successful ECT (Sackeim *et al*, 1990), and further research is required to identify the most appropriate pharmacological treatment for the continuation and maintenance phases of treatment. For all patients, the first four months after successful ECT is the time of highest risk of relapse, and this should influence the arrangements for psychiatric supervision.

Recommendations

(1) The best predictor of a good response to ECT is the number of the typical features of depressive illness.
(2) ECT may be particularly effective in depressive illness with psychotic features.
(3) Depressed patients who have not responded to antidepressant drug treatment may recover if treated subsequently by ECT.
(4) Continuation antidepressant drug treatment is essential after successful ECT.

References

ABRAMS, R. (1992) *Electroconvulsive Therapy* (2nd edn) Oxford: Oxford University Press.
AMERICAN PSYCHIATRIC ASSOCIATION (1990) *The Practice of Electroconvulsive Therapy: Recommendations for Treatment, Training and Privileging.* Washington, DC: American Psychiatric Association.
BARTON, J. L., MEHTA, S. & SNAITH, R. P. (1973) Prophylactic value of ECT in depressive illness. *Acta Psychiatrica Scandinavica,* **49**, 386–392.
BRANDON, S., COWLEY, P., MCDONALD, C., *et al* (1984) Electroconvulsive therapy – results in depressive illness from the Leicestershire trial. *British Medical Journal,* **288**, 23–25.

BUCHAN, H., JOHNSTONE, E. C., McPHERSON, K., *et al* (1992) Who benefits from electroconvulsive therapy? Combined results of the Leicester and Northwick Park trials. *British Journal of Psychiatry*, **160**, 355–359.

COFFEY, C. E., WEINER, R. D., DJANG, W. T., *et al* (1991) Brain anatomic effects of electroconvulsive therapy. *Archives of General Psychiatry*, **48**, 1013–1021.

FREEMAN, C. P. L., BASSON, J. V. & CRICHTON, A. (1978) Double-blind controlled trial of electroconvulsive therapy (ECT) and simulated ECT in depressive illness. *Lancet*, i, 738–740.

GANGADHAR, B. N., KAPUR, R. L. & KALYANASUNDARAM, S. (1982) Comparison of electroconvulsive therapy with imipramine in endogenous depression – a double blind study. *British Journal of Psychiatry*, **141**, 367–371.

——, JANAKIRAMAIAH, N., SUBBAKRISHNA, D. K., *et al* (1993) Twice versus thrice weekly ECT in melancholia – a double-blind prospective comparison. *Journal of Affective Disorders*, **27**, 273–278.

GREENBLATT, M., GROSSER, G. H. & WECHSLER, H. (1964) Differential response of hospitalised depressed patients in somatic therapy. *American Journal of Psychiatry*, **120**, 935–943.

GREGORY, S., SAWCROSS, C. R. & GILL, D. (1985) The Nottingham ECT study – a double blind comparison of bilateral, unilateral and simulated ECT in depressive illness. *British Journal of Psychiatry*, **146**, 520–524.

JOHNSTONE, E. C., DEAKIN, J. F. W., LAWLEY, P., *et al* (1980) The Northwick Park ECT trial. *Lancet*, ii, 1317–1320.

McALLISTER, D. A., PERRI, M. G., JORDAN, R. C., *et al* (1987) The effects of ECT given two versus three times weekly. *Psychiatry Research*, **21**, 63–69.

MEDICAL RESEARCH COUNCIL (1965) Chemical trial of the treatment of depressive illness. *British Medical Journal*, i, 881–886.

PIPPARD, J. & ELLAM, L. (1981) *Electroconvulsive Treatment in Great Britain, 1980*. London: Gaskell.

PRUDIC, J., SACKEIM, H. A. & DEVANAND, D. P. (1990) Medication resistance and clinical response to electroconvulsive therapy. *Psychiatry Research*, **31**, 287–296.

RODGER, C. R., SCOTT, A. I. F. & WHALLEY, L. J. (1994) Is there a delay in the onset of the antidepressant effect of electroconvulsive therapy? *British Journal of Psychiatry*, **164**, 106–109.

ROYAL COLLEGE OF PSYCHIATRISTS (1977) Memorandum on the use of electroconvulsive therapy. *British Journal of Psychiatry*, **131**, 261–272.

SACKEIM, H. A., PRUDIC, J., DEVANAND, D. P., *et al* (1990) The impact of medication resistance and continuation pharmacotherapy on relapse following response to electroconvulsive therapy in major depression. *Journal of Clinical Psychopharmacology*, **10**, 96–104.

SCOTT, A. I. F. (1989) Which depressed patients will respond to electroconvulsive therapy? *British Journal of Psychiatry*, **154**, 8–17.

——, TURNBULL, L. W., BLANE, A., *et al* (1991) Electroconvulsive therapy and brain damage. *Lancet*, **338**, 264.

—— & WHALLEY, L. J. (1993) The onset and rate of the antidepressant effect of electroconvulsive therapy – a neglected topic of research. *British Journal of Psychiatry*, **162**, 725–732.

STRÖMGREN, L. S. (1975) Therapeutic results in brief interval unilateral ECT. *Acta Psychiatrica Scandinavica*, **52**, 246–255.

WEST, E. (1981) Electroconvulsive therapy in depression – a double-blind controlled trial. *British Medical Journal*, **282**, 355–357.

2. ECT in mania

J. Pippard

ECT has long been known to be an effective treatment for manic excitement, both from many reports from the 1940s and 1950s and in general clinical experience. The success of antipsychotic drugs and lithium has reduced the use of ECT in mania, but in both the US (Consensus Conference, 1985) and UK (Pippard & Ellam, 1981) about 2–3% of patients receiving ECT are given it for mania.

Until 1988 there had been no controlled trials, but several retrospective studies. A recent retrospective chart review (Black *et al*, 1987) of 438 manic patients, covering 12 years to 1981, compared ECT, adequate and inadequate lithium, and neither ECT nor lithium; most patients were given antipsychotic medication. A significantly greater number (78%) who had ECT showed "marked improvement" than did the 62% who had adequate lithium treatment or the 37% given neither. Twelve of 16 patients (75%) who failed to respond to adequate lithium markedly improved with ECT.

In the only prospective comparison of ECT with lithium (Small *et al*, 1988), 34 manic patients were randomly allocated to treatment with either lithium or an average series of nine bilateral ECT treatments at a frequency of three per week (the first six patients randomised to ECT were given unilateral treatment with little or no benefit until changed to bilateral treatment and this was used on all subsequent patients). No patient on ECT was given lithium until the end of the eight-week trial period, but more than half of the patients in both groups received neuroleptics in the lowest possible dosage, for example, for control of psychosis or dangerous behaviour. During the first eight weeks of treatment, ratings on a number of scales uniformly and significantly favoured the ECT group. The improvement, rated by non-blind research nurses and a clinician, was confirmed by blind ratings of videotapes by an independent psychiatrist. After eight weeks there were no significant group differences. The conclusion was that an average series of nine bilateral ECT followed by maintenance lithium is a useful alternative to lithium, with likely short-term advantages for ECT, particularly in patients with mixed manic and depressive symptoms or very severe manic states. Subsequent rates of relapse, recurrence and readmission to hospital were comparable.

Many clinicians believe that ECT needs to be given more intensively in treating mania than for other conditions, but there is no clear agreement about this. In the past it was sometimes given twice daily for one to two days to bring about rapid subsidence of severe excitement. Taylor (1982) recommended bilateral ECT daily at first. Some reports have found no difference between unilateral and bilateral ECT, but no controlled comparisons have been made and unless there are strong indications for using unilateral ECT, it is advisable to give bilateral treatment and to consider more frequent application than the usual twice-weekly British regime.

Recommendations

(1) ECT may in occasional circumstances be the treatment of choice for severely manic patients.

(2) ECT may be a safe alternative to high-dose neuroleptics, with the advantage of a faster therapeutic response.

(3) ECT should be considered in less disturbed manic patients with slow or inadequate response to medication.

(4) The clinical state of the patient may mean that ECT has to be delivered on the ward rather than in an ECT suite.

References

BLACK, D. W., WINOKUR, G. & NASRALLAH, A. (1987) A naturalistic study of ECT versus lithium in 438 patients. *Journal of Clinical Psychiatry,* **48**, 132–139.

CONSENSUS CONFERENCE: ECT (1985) *Journal of the American Medical Association,* **254**, 2103–2108.

PIPPARD, J. & ELLAM, L. (1981) *ECT in Great Britain, 1980.* London: Gaskell.

SMALL, J. G., KLAPPER, M. H., KELLAMS, J. J., *et al* (1988) ECT compared with lithium in the management of manic states. *Archives of General Psychiatry,* **45**, 727–732.

TAYLOR, M. A. (1982) Indications for electroconvulsive treatment. In *ECT: Biological Foundations and Clinical Applications* (eds R. Abrams & W. B. Essman). New York: SP Medical Scientific Books.

3. ECT in schizophrenia

T. Lock

Growing concern about the side-effects of neuroleptic drugs and high-dose treatment regimes has prompted a reappraisal of the role of ECT in schizophrenia.

Before the introduction of neuroleptic drugs, insulin comas, alone or combined with ECT, or ECT on its own were the main somatic treatments for schizophrenia, and it was widely believed that between 12 and 20 treatments were needed to ensure a therapeutic response. Early open-trial (May, 1968) and placebo-controlled studies (Miller *et al*, 1953; Ulett *et al*, 1956; Brill *et al*,1959; Heath *et al*, 1964) are flawed by a variety of methodological errors and are difficult to interpret, while more recent single-blind (Janakiramaiah *et al*, 1982) and double-blind (Taylor & Fleminger, 1980; Brandon *et al*, 1985; Abraham & Kulhara, 1987) trials of ECT in schizophrenia have incorporated concurrent neuroleptic treatment in their research design. There is, nevertheless, some consistency about the results which suggest that ECT does have a role in the treatment of some patients with a primary diagnosis of schizophrenia. Schizophrenia is not, however, a homogeneous disorder and it is necessary to define which patient subgroups are likely to benefit from ECT. The current concept of the disorder, in terms of symptom patterns and therapeutic responsiveness, is that of two fairly distinct groups: Type I, characterised by 'positive' (florid) symptoms which tend to respond well to neuroleptics; and Type II, the so-called 'defect' state, characterised by negative symptoms such as affective flattening and poverty of speech and drive, which respond poorly, if at all, to neuroleptic medication. The concept of 'drug-resistant' schizophrenia is extremely vague, as it may be applicable to both the above subgroups.

Type II

There is no evidence to suggest that ECT is effective in the treatment of patients with Type II symptoms *per se* (Miller *et al*, 1953; Brill *et al*, 1959; Heath *et al*, 1964), although marked depressive symptoms arising in the context of a Type II syndrome may respond to ECT.

Type I

Several studies have demonstrated that ECT is effective, in terms of symptomatic relief, length of hospitalisation and discharge rate, in the treatment of Type I patients (Ulett *et al*, 1956; May, 1968; Folstein *et al*, 1973; Taylor & Fleminger, 1980; Janakiramaiah *et al*, 1982; Koehler & Sauer, 1983; Brandon *et al*, 1985; Abraham & Kulhara, 1987). May (1968), in his 228 patient study, demonstrated that ECT (on its own) was effective in the treatment of Type I patients, but less effective than phenothiazines. Taylor & Fleminger (1980), Brandon *et al* (1985) and Abraham & Kulhara (1987) used a similar research method to compare the effects of augmenting low (that is, less than 500 mg/day) chlorpromazine with real versus sham ECT; their findings were consistent. Taken together, a total of 59 Type I patients were treated (30 with real ECT-plus-drug and 29 with sham ECT-plus-drug). The number of treatments given in these studies was 12 or less. Both patient groups showed a significant symptomatic improvement over the study period, but patients treated with real ECT responded significantly faster than those treated with sham ECT for the first four weeks (i.e. during the time that real/sham ECT was being delivered). The sham ECT patients then began to catch up, and, by about 8–12 weeks there was no significant difference in the symptomatic ratings of the real and sham ECT patients. Additionally, there was evidence that some patients who responded well to the real ECT-plus-drug regimen experienced a relapse of symptoms when ECT was discontinued (see Taylor, 1990), and it is possible that these patients would have sustained their initial symptomatic improvement had a longer course of ECT been administered. Janakiramaiah *et al* (1982) compared the efficacy of ECT given in combination with either low-dose (300 mg daily) or high-dose (500 mg daily) chlorpromazine. A therapeutic advantage was demonstrated for the low-dose group, but there was no advantage in administering ECT to patients already receiving high doses of chlorpromazine. The effect of ECT in combination with other neuroleptics is unknown, but it seems reasonable to assume that the same principles would apply to low and high dose equivalents of other neuroleptics.

Contrary to expectations, both schizophrenic-type and depressive-type symptoms respond to ECT (Taylor & Fleminger, 1980; Brandon *et al*, 1985). Type I symptoms which respond to ECT include passivity, persecutory delusions, delusional mood, thought interference, and associated depressive symptoms. Predictors of good outcome include depressive features, short duration of illness or episode, and absence of premorbid schizoid or paranoid traits (Dodwell & Goldberg, 1989).

Although definitive evidence is lacking, clinical case studies confirm the effectiveness of ECT in specific Type I subgroups, particularly when psychotic symptoms are found in association with intercurrent affective symptoms and/or alterations of motor behaviour:

(1) acute catatonic states (catatonic excitement or immobility);
(2) schizoaffective disorders;
(3) acute drug-induced schizophreniform disorders (e.g. dopaminomimetic psychosis in Parkinson's disease, phencyclidine psychosis);
(4) acute paranoid syndromes;
(5) patients with neuroleptic malignant syndrome (see ECT in NMS).

ECT has no place in the management of violent or offending behaviour as such. The most common link between antisocial behaviour and psychosis is between violence and schizophrenia presenting with delusional symptoms (Taylor *et al*, in press). An early study (Smith *et al*, 1967) noted that schizophrenics with symptoms of hostility and persecutory delusions responded favourably to a combination of ECT and neuroleptics. Given that some acutely ill schizophrenic patients in a forensic setting fail to respond to high doses of neuroleptic medication and/or tolerate neuroleptic medication poorly, ECT may have a limited role in the symptomatic management of patients whose hostility is clearly a response to an underlying Type I psychosis.

No research has been undertaken comparing the efficacy of maintenance ECT versus maintenance neuroleptic medication.

Recommendations

(1) ECT is not recommended for Type II schizophrenic patients; the exception is when marked depressive symptoms arise in the context of a Type II syndrome.
(2) The practical usefulness of ECT in type I schizophrenic patients is limited to patients:
    (a) who are unable to tolerate a dose of a neuroleptic equivalent to 500 mg chlorpromazine daily;
    (b) who are responding poorly to a dose of a neuroleptic equivalent to 500 mg chlorpromazine daily;
    (c) where the maximum rate of symptomatic response is required;
    (d) specific subgroups (see above).
(3) ECT may reduce antisocial behaviour which occurs as a response to underlying Type I psychotic symptoms when antipsychotic medication alone fails to alleviate psychotic symptoms.

References

ABRAHAM, K. R. & KULHARA, P. (1987) The efficacy of electroconvulsive therapy in the treatment of schizophrenia. *British Journal of Psychiatry*, **151**, 152–155.

BRANDON, S., COWLEY, P., McDONALD, C., *et al* (1985) Leicester ECT trial – results in schizophrenia. *British Journal of Psychiatry*, **146**, 177–183.

BRILL, N. Q., CRUMPTON, E., EIDUSON, S., *et al* (1959) Relative effectiveness of various components of electroconvulsive therapy. *Archives of Neurology and Psychiatry*, **81**, 627–635.

DODWELL, D. & GOLDBERG, D. (1989) A study of factors associated with response to electroconvulsive therapy in patients with schizophrenic symptoms. *British Journal of Psychiatry*, **154**, 635–639.

FOLSTEIN, M., FOLSTEIN, S. & McHUGH, P. R. (1973) Clinical predictors of improvement after electroconvulsive therapy for schizophrenia, neurotic reactions and affective disorder. *Biological Psychiatry*, **7**, 147–152.

HEATH, E. S., ADAMS, A. & WAKELING, P. L. G. (1964) Short courses of ECT and simulated ECT in chronic schizophrenia. *British Journal of Psychiatry*, **110**, 800–807.

JANAKIRAMAIAH, N., CHANNABASAVANNA, S. M., NARASIMHA-MURTHY, N. S. (1982) ECT/chlorpromazine combination versus chlorpromazine alone in acutely schizophrenic patients. *Acta Psychiatrica Scandinavica*, **66**, 464–470.

KOEHLER, K. & SAUER, H. (1983) First rank symptoms as predictors of ECT response in schizophrenia. *British Journal of Psychiatry*, **142**, 280–283.

MAY, P. R. A. (1968) *Treatment of Schizophrenia*. New York: Science House.

MILLER, D. H., CLANCY, J. & CUMMING, E. (1953) A comparison between unidirectional current nonconvulsive electrical stimulation given with a Reiter's machine, standard alternating current electroshock and pentothal in chronic schizophrenia. *American Journal of Psychiatry*, **109**, 617–620.

SMITH, K., SURPHLIS, W. R. P., GYNTHER, M. D., *et al* (1967) ECT-chlorpromazine and chlorpromazine compared in the treatment of schizophrenia. *Journal of Nervous and Mental Disease*, **144**, 284–290.

TAYLOR, P. J. (1990) Schizophrenia and ECT – a case for change in prescription? In *Dilemmas and Difficulties in the Management of Psychiatric Patients* (eds K. Hawton & P. Cowan). Oxford: Oxford University Press.

—— & FLEMINGER, J. J. (1980) ECT for schizophrenia. *Lancet*, **i**, 1380–1382.

——, MULLEN, P. & WESSLEY, S. (1995) Psychosis, violence and crime. In *Forensic Psychiatry: Clinical, Legal and Ethical Issues* (eds J. Gunn & P. J. Taylor). Oxford: Heinemann-Butterworth (in press).

ULETT, G. A., SMITH, K. & GLESER, G. C. (1956) Evaluation of convulsive and subconvulsive shock therapies utilising a control group. *American Journal of Psychiatry*, **112**, 795–802.

4. ECT as a specific treatment for neuropsychiatric conditions

T. Lock & R. McClelland

Catatonia

The prevalence of catatonia has markedly declined in the Western world since the introduction of effective psychotropic agents, but cases are still reported in the developing world. Catatonia is now thought to be closely related to bipolar affective disorders, although catatonic symptoms (excitement, stupor, mutism, negativism, posturing and rigidity) may occur as a complication of a variety of functional and organic psychiatric illnesses.

The extreme form, described as lethal catatonia (LC), may present with muscle rigidity, mutism, fluctuating level of consciousness, hyperpyrexia, autonomic instability, haematological and biochemical abnormalities, and may lead to dehydration, exhaustion and death if left untreated (Mann *et al*, 1986). The full-blown clinical presentation is symptomatically indistinguishable from the neuroleptic malignant syndrome (NMS), a side-effect of neuroleptic agents, or malignant hyperthermia (MH), a rare complication of general anaesthesia (Mann *et al*, 1986; Kellam, 1987; White & Robins, 1991). It is important to distinguish between catatonia and NMS, for catatonia is potentially responsive to neuroleptics, whereas neuroleptics should be discontinued in cases of NMS. The differential diagnosis is dependent on a reliable medication history and a description of the temporal sequence of events leading up to the full-blown syndrome. White & Robins (1991), working in a developing country, pointed out, however, that the distinction between catatonia and NMS is quite arbitrary in some cases – for example, separate episodes of catatonia and NMS occurred in one patient (White, 1992).

There have been no double-blind trials of ECT in catatonic states, but a number of case reports suggest that ECT is a particularly effective form of treatment (Abrams & Essman, 1982).

Recommendations

(1) ECT is an effective form of treatment in catatonic states, and may be life-saving in cases of lethal catatonia.
(2) ECT may have a potentially life-saving role in the treatment of cases where the differential diagnosis of NMS and LC is unclear.

References

ABRAMS, R. & ESSMAN, W. B. (eds) (1982) *Electroconvulsive Therapy – Biological Foundations and Clinical Applications.* New York: SP Medical and Scientific Books.

KELLAM, A. M. P. (1987) The neuroleptic malignant syndrome, so called – a survey of the world literature. *British Journal of Psychiatry*, **150**, 752–759.

MANN, S. C., CAROFF, S. N., BLEIER, H. R., *et al* (1986) Lethal catatonia. *American Journal of Psychiatry*, **143**, 1374–1381.

WHITE, D. A. C. (1992) Catatonia and the neuroleptic malignant syndrome – a single entity? *British Journal of Psychiatry*, **161**, 558–560.

—— & ROBINS, A. H. (1991) Catatonia – harbinger of the neuroleptic malignant syndrome? *British Journal of Psychiatry*, **158**, 419–421.

Parkinson's disease

Parkinson's disease, which affects 1% of the population over 50, is commonly associated with depression. Several case studies have reported improvements not only in depression, but in Parkinsonian symptoms following ECT. The question has therefore been raised of whether or not ECT may have a direct therapeutic effect in Parkinson's disease.

The most authoritative study to date has been a double-blind investigation of non-depressed patients with Parkinson's disease with the 'on-off' syndrome (Anderson *et al*, 1987). This study confirmed earlier observations that ECT has an anti-Parkinsonian effect in drug-resistant patients. Predictors of a good response were older age at the time of treatment and longer duration of L-dopa therapy. The duration of the response to ECT appears to be very variable and in most cases relatively short-lived, lasting weeks only. It is possible that maintenance ECT may offer longer lasting symptomatic improvements. The place of ECT in Parkinson's disease probably awaits the results of more authoritative prospective studies (Fink, 1988). The efficacy of ECT in some patients with Parkinson's disease is further evidence that ECT affects dopamine receptor sensitivity, a mechanism which seems likely to underpin its therapeutic efficacy in severe depression.

Recommendations

(1)   ECT has a short-term anti-Parkinsonian effect.
(2)   The place of maintenance ECT in Parkinson's disease has not been established.

References

ANDERSON, K., BALLDIN, J., GOTTFIRES, C. G., *et al* (1987) A double-blind evaluation of electroconvulsive therapy in Parkinson's disease with 'on-off' phenomena. *Acta Neurologica Scandinavica*, **76**, 191–199.
FINK, M. (1988) ECT for Parkinson's disease? *Convulsive Therapy*, 189–191.

Neuroleptic malignant syndrome (NMS)

NMS is characterised by muscle rigidity, mutism, fluctuating level of consciousness, hyperpyrexia, autonomic instability and haematological and biochemical abnormalities, and may lead to dehydration, exhaustion, respiratory and renal failure and death if left untreated. The mortality rate may be as high as 24% (Kellam, 1987; Davis *et al*, 1991). The syndrome is clinically indistinguishable from malignant hyperthermia (MH), a rare complication of general anaesthesia, and lethal catatonia (LC), which may occur as a complication of functional and organic psychiatric illness *per se*. The diagnosis of NMS is dependent on a reliable medication history and a description of the temporal sequence of events leading up to the full blown syndrome, and is notoriously difficult (White, 1992): NMS may be obscured by a coexistent infective illness, and may be precipitated by dehydration or physical exhaustion in patients already on neuroleptic medication (Renwick *et al*, 1992). NMS and MH can be distinguished by the response to muscle relaxants, but the distinction between NMS and LC can be quite arbitrary in some cases.

The current approach to the management of NMS includes immediate withdrawal of neuroleptic drugs, rehydration and intensive monitoring. No consensus exists as to what to do if the above measures fail to reverse symptoms. Treatment with drugs which act either centrally (such as bromocriptine) or peripherally (such as dantrolene) to decrease muscle contraction has been shown to be more successful than supportive treatment alone (Rosenberg & Green, 1989). Both bromocriptine and dantrolene appear to have a mean response time of less or equal to 48 hours. Other drugs used in the treatment of NMS include amantadine, L-dopa, steroids, benzodiazepines, and anticholinergics. The mortality rate is about 9.7% if patients are treated with 'specific' drugs, and 10.3% if patients are treated with ECT (Davis *et al*, 1991). There have been no double-blind trials of any 'specific' treatment approaches, and the relative efficacy and safety of these treatments is unknown.

The rationale for using ECT as a 'specific' treatment for NMS is based on its efficacy in treating LC and bipolar affective disorders associated with catatonic symptoms. ECT may have a potentially life-saving role in the treatment of cases where the differential diagnosis of NMS and LC is unclear (Addonizio & Susman, 1987).

Thirty-one cases have been reported where ECT was used as a 'specific' treatment for NMS where the diagnosis of the syndrome was certain (Addonizio & Susman, 1987; Harland *et al*, 1990; Scheftner & Shulman, 1992). ECT was used as a 'first line' treatment (preceded by supportive therapy only) in 16 cases, and in conjunction with or preceded by 'specific' drug therapy in 15 cases, and was associated with a good overall outcome in 85% of the patients. A symptomatic response (that is, a sustained decrease in temperature and/or muscle rigidity) was observed within 0.5 to four hours after the first ECT in five patients; within 24 hours in ten; and within 72 hours in four. The response time of the remaining six 'good outcome' cases is unknown. These figures suggest that an immediate (that is, within 24 hours) symptomatic improvement can be expected in about 50% of cases, and that at least 60% will respond to ECT within 72 hours. ECT was effective in eight out of nine patients who had apparently failed to respond to dantrolene or bromocriptine (on their own, in combination, and/or in conjunction with steroids, benzodiazepines or anticholinergics), and four cases previously treated with steroids, benzodiazepines or anticholinergics (on their own, or in combination).

The subtle effect of literature bias (that is, cases with a successful outcome are more likely to be published than cases with an equivocal outcome) may be contributing to the apparent efficacy of ECT in cases of NMS. Furthermore, the diagnosis of NMS was made retrospectively in some of these patients, and alternative 'specific' drug therapy, which may have been more practical and equally effective as a first line intervention, was not tried in 13 'good outcome' cases.

ECT was associated with a poor outcome in 15% of the 31 cases: one patient showed an equivocal clinical response, but no untoward side-effects; one patient had a cardiac arrest but suffered no sequelae after resuscitation and was successfully treated with ECT a year later for a psychotic depressive illness; one patient developed permanent brain damage after a cardiac arrest; and two patients died (one following a cardiac arrest). ECT could not, however, be singled out as the primary cause of the disasters; furthermore, neuroleptic medication was not discontinued in the three patients with disastrous outcomes.

Autonomic instability is characteristic of NMS (and LC) and patients with NMS may be particularly vulnerable to developing cardiac arrhythmias with ECT. Brief atrial arrhythmias were reported in at least two of the 31 cases in addition to the three patients who suffered cardiac arrests. Certain muscle relaxants (for example, succinylcholine) may precipitate hyperkalaemia in patients with significant muscle damage, and this may add to the risk of cardiac arrhythmia in patients with acute NMS (Liskow, 1985).

Evidence of psychosis is likely to reappear during or soon after resolution of the acute NMS episode. Six studies have reported on the efficacy of ECT as an alternative to neuroleptic medication, or in combination with low-dose thioridazine, in the treatment of psychotic patients who have recovered from an acute NMS (Adityanjee *et al*, 1989). Patients with NMS do not appear to be at increased risk of developing MH as a complication of anaesthesia after the acute NMS has resolved (Hermesh *et al*, 1988).

Recommendations

(1) Patients with suspected NMS require immediate discontinuation of neuroleptic medication, intensive monitoring and supportive therapy; the latter is best provided in an intensive therapy unit (ITU).

(2) If a specific treatment is required, dantrolene and/or bromocriptine should be used first in most cases, for both drugs have been shown to be effective, and drug therapy can usually be initiated more promptly than ECT in most ITU settings.

(3) ECT may be the treatment of first choice in severe cases as it acts more rapidly than dantrolene or bromocriptine.

(4) ECT may be useful in patients who have not responded to adequate drug treatment within 48 hours.

(5) The administration of ECT to a patient with acute or subacute NMS should be by experienced ECT staff and in the ITU. Succinylcholine should not be used as the muscle relaxant; serum potassium levels and the electrocardiogram require particularly close observation.

(6) ECT may be useful in the management of psychotic patients after the acute episode and where there appears to be a significant risk of recurrence of NMS were neuroleptics to be recommenced.

(7) ECT may have a potentially life-saving role in the treatment of cases where the differential diagnosis of NMS and LC is unclear.

References

ADDONIZIO, G. & SUSMAN, V. L. (1987) ECT as a treatment alternative for patients with symptoms of neuroleptic malignant syndrome. *Journal of Clinical Psychiatry*, **48**, 102–105.

ADITYANJEE, D. A. S., DITYANJEE, P. & CHAWLA, H. M. (1989) Neuroleptic malignant syndrome and psychosis. *British Journal of Psychiatry*, **155**, 852–854.

DAVIS, J. M., JANICAK, P. G., SAKKAS, P., *et al* (1991) Electroconvulsive therapy in the treatment of the neuroleptic malignant syndrome. *Convulsive Therapy*, **7**, 111–120.

HARLAND, C. C., O'LEARY, M. M., WINTERS, R., *et al* (1990) Neuroleptic malignant syndrome: a case for electroconvulsive therapy. *Postgraduate Medical Journal*, **66**, 49-51.

HERMESH, H., AIZENBERG, D., LAPIDOT, M., *et al* (1988) Risk of malignant hyperthermia among patients with neuroleptic malignant syndrome and their families. *American Journal of Psychiatry*, **145**, 1431–1434.

KELLAM, A. M. P. (1987) The neuroleptic malignant syndrome, so called – a survey of the literature. *British Journal of Psychiatry*, **150**, 752–759.

LISKOW, B. I. (1985) Relationship between neuroleptic malignant syndrome and malignant hyperthermia. *American Journal of Psychiatry*, **142**, 390.

RENWICK, D. R., CHANDRAKER, A. & BANNISTER, P. (1992) Missed neuroleptic malignant syndrome. *British Medical Journal*, **304**, 831–832.

ROSENBERG, N. R. & GREEN, M. (1989) Neuroleptic malignant syndrome: review of response to therapy. *Archives of Internal Medicine*, **149**, 1927–1931.

SCHEFTNER, W. A. & SHULMAN, R. B. (1992) Treatment choice in neuroleptic malignant syndrome. *Convulsive Therapy*, **8**, 267–279.

WHITE, D. A. C. (1992) Catatonia and the neuroleptic malignant syndrome – a single entity? *British Journal of Psychiatry*, **161**, 158.

Drug-induced extrapyramidal syndromes

Goswami *et al* (1989) demonstrated that schizophrenic patients with acute Parkinsonian side-effects to neuroleptic medication had significantly fewer extrapyramidal symptoms when treated with an ECT–procyclidine–neuroleptic combination than patients treated with procyclidine–neuroleptic alone. Unfortunately, minimal reference was made to psychotic symptoms, and the dose of procyclidine was not stated, so it is possible that an increased dose of procyclidine might have been equally effective. Furthermore, the advantage offered by ECT only lasted a week.

Adityanjee *et al* (1990) described the effects of ECT in one patient with florid psychotic symptoms whose neuroleptic medication had been discontinued because of disabling tardive extrapyramidal side-effects (severe torticollis). They noted that the florid psychotic symptoms had improved by the fourth ECT, and that the dystonia was also starting to improve significantly by the eleventh ECT, but it had started to worsen again two months after ECT.

Recommendations

(1) The role of ECT in the treatment of neuroleptic-induced extrapyramidal side-effects remains to be established.
(2) ECT has a limited role in that it may ameliorate suffering in the short-term, but with little likelihood of producing a sustained resolution of symptoms.

References

ADITYANJEE JAYASWAL, S. K., CHAN, T. M. & SUBRAMANIAM, M. (1990) Temporary remission of tardive dystonia following ECT. *British Journal of Psychiatry,* **156**, 433–435.
GOSWAMI, U., DUTTA, S., KURUVILLA, K., *et al* (1989) Electroconvulsive therapy in neuroleptic-induced Parkinsonism. *Biological Psychiatry,* **26**, 234–238.

Epilepsy and related disorders

ECT is a powerful anticonvulsant, as demonstrated by an average rise in seizure threshold of 80% (range 25–200 %) during a course of ECT (Kalinowski & Kennedy, 1943; Sackeim *et al*, 1987; see also Chapter 22). There have been no open or controlled studies comparing ECT with conventional anti-epileptic drugs for the treatment of spontaneous seizure disorders *per se*, but several case studies have been reported which suggest that ECT is an effective anti-epileptic treatment.

In most of these studies, ECT was used to treat a variety of mental disturbances associated with spontaneous seizure disorders (Kalinowski & Kennedy, 1943; Caplan, 1946; Schnur *et al*, 1989). Taken together, ECT appears to be very effective at terminating the more acute types of mental disturbance which are thought to be directly related to underlying (spontaneous) seizure activity, such as ictal, fugue and twilight states and post-ictal acute organic brain syndromes (e.g. delirium). In these conditions, a single ECT treatment may be effective. The aetiological relationship between the more chronic disorders associated with epilepsy (e.g. affective, paranoid and schizophreniform psychoses) and the underlying seizure disorder is less direct, and the efficacy of ECT with respect to treating these disorders is similar to when ECT is used to treat similar disorders in non-epileptic patients. In Schnur's study of five patients with the syndrome of episodic aggressive dyscontrol (Schnur *et al*, 1989), a course of 9 to 14 (mean 10.8) ECT treatments – using contemporary machines and a contemporary administration technique – induced a complete remission of aggressive episodes in four out of five patients during the course of treatment, and a complete remission in the incidence of spontaneous seizures.

Similar findings were reported in the older studies (Kalinowski & Kennedy, 1943; Caplan, 1946). Not only was ECT effective in the treatment of the mental state disturbances for which it was administered, but it also brought about a complete remission of spontaneous seizures during the course of treatment in a large majority of patients. This effect was, however, short-lived, and the frequency of spontaneous seizures was noted to return to baseline pre-ECT levels within the two month period after discontinuation of ECT. Continuation (maintenance) ECT (e.g. one treatment every 7–10 days) however, had a more sustained anti-epileptic effect in that the frequency of spontaneous seizures was reduced by about 60% on average compared with baseline levels. Sackeim *et al* (1983) reported on a critically ill patient who was treated with ECT in a somewhat desperate attempt to terminate generalised status epilepticus which had failed to respond to a variety of potent intravenous anticonvulsant drugs. Two ECT treatments were given, and were effective in terminating the episode of status, but the patient later died.

Recommendations

(1) ECT is very effective at terminating the acute mental state disturbances associated with spontaneous seizures which appear to have a direct relationship to the underlying

seizure disorder, e.g. fugue, twilight, and post-ictal confusional states. One or a small number of ECT treatments may suffice.

(2)   ECT is effective in the treatment of other more chronic mental state disturbances which are encountered in epileptic patients, e.g. schizophreniform and affective psychoses. Spontaneous epilepsy is neither a contraindication nor a specific reason for using ECT to treat a coexistent mental state disorder in an epileptic patient.

(3)   ECT is a powerful anticonvulsant treatment, but the anticonvulsant effect is dependent on ongoing ECT applications. Given the efficacy of contemporary anti-epileptic drugs, ECT is only likely to be considered as a viable anti-convulsant treatment option in desperate cases where conventional drug treatment has failed.

References

CAPLAN, G. (1946) Electrical convulsion therapy in the treatment of epilepsy. *Journal of Mental Science,* **92,** 784–793.

KALINOWSKI, L. B. & KENNEDY, F. (1943) Observations in electric shock therapy applied to problems of epilepsy. *Electric Shock Therapy and Epilepsy,* 56–67.

SACKEIM, H. A., DECINA, P., PROHOVNIK, I., *et al* (1983) Anticonvulsant and antidepressant properties of electroconvulsive therapy: A proposed mechanism of action. *Biological Psychiatry,* **18,** 1301–1310.

——, ——, ——, *et al* (1987) Seizure threshold in electroconvulsive therapy. *Archives of General Psychiatry,* **44,** 355–360.

SCHNUR, D. B., MUKHERJEE, S., SILVER, J., *et al* (1989) ECT in the treatment of episodic aggressive dyscontrol in psychotic patients. *Convulsive Therapy,* 353–361.

5. ECT in the elderly patient

S. M. Benbow

Age is not a contraindication to the use of ECT. A number of studies over the years have found that increasing age predicts a favourable treatment response. Reviewers have concluded that elderly people respond at least as well to ECT as younger people do. Nevertheless, when ECT is to be prescribed for an elderly person some age-related factors need consideration.

Physical illness may coexist in elderly patients referred for ECT and will need careful assessment before treatment. Cardiovascular disease is a particular concern and this group of patients are at increased risk of developing complications during treatment.

Some older patients are more likely to have memory difficulties and acute confusion during ECT. Careful repeated assessment of their cognitive function and response to treatment will therefore be important as the course of treatment proceeds. A standardised instrument for monitoring cognitive function is useful. Attention will need to be paid to measures which minimise the adverse cognitive effects of treatment, such as electrode placement, treatment frequency, stimulus intensity, concurrent medication, and so on. The clinical practice of many clinicians, having minimised any factors contributing to confusion during treatment, is to continue treatment despite the confusional state and to expect it to subside when treatment has been discontinued, although sometimes not for four to eight weeks (Summers *et al*, 1979).

Since seizure threshold may rise with increasing age (Sackeim *et al*, 1987), close attention will need to be paid to factors which may affect seizure threshold, such as concurrent drug treatments, dose of anaesthetic drugs and adequate ventilation. Seizure augmentation may need consideration if duration of seizures remains short despite minimising any contributory factors, unless clinical improvement is satisfactory.

Recommendations

(1) ECT may be the treatment of choice for depressive illness.
(2) Treatment is not contraindicated by age alone.
(3) Take special care with concomitant medication and with the physical assessment of patients prior to ECT.
(4) The seizure threshold may be relatively high in some elderly patients and these patients may require a relatively high stimulus charge.
(5) Special precautions may be needed to guard against memory impairment or confusion (for example, longer gaps between each treatment).

References

SACKEIM, H. A., DECINA, P., PORTNOY, S., *et al* (1987) Studies of dosage, seizure threshold and seizure duration in ECT. *Biological Psychiatry*, **22**, 249–268.

SUMMERS, W. K., ROBINS, E. & REICH, T. (1979) The natural history of acute organic mental syndrome after bilateral electroconvulsive therapy. *Biological Psychiatry*, **14**, 905–912.

6. ECT in those under 18 years old

C. P. Freeman

This section deals specifically with ECT in those individuals who are 17 years old or less. The comments below should be seen as additional to those in the rest of the guidelines. All the points made about the good practice of ECT in the rest of this document apply to those under the age of 18. Although ECT is very rarely administered to children and young people, we have produced separate notes for this age group primarily because we are aware of the considerable debate there is about the use of "ECT in children" and the recommendation from some groups such as MIND that "ECT in children" should be banned.

Indications for ECT in young people aged 13–17

These are essentially the same as for patients who are 18 years and over. The disorders for which ECT is indicated in adults often have their onset in childhood and adolescence. Severe major depressive illness, bipolar disorder and schizophrenia can begin and recur during childhood or adolescence. Just as in adulthood, these disorders can be resistant to other forms of treatment such as psychotherapy, family therapy and antidepressant drugs. They can also be as severe as adult disorders and be associated with a considerable risk of self-harm, either through suicidal behaviour or because of inability or refusal to eat and drink. In these circumstances ECT can be life-saving.

Just as in adults, major depression presenting in childhood and adolescence may develop without any obvious antecedents such as losses, major life stresses and interpersonal difficulties, or it may be precipitated by anything from quite minor to overwhelming life events. It is the clinical features of the depression rather than its understandability in psychological terms which should determine whether treatments such as antidepressant drugs and/or ECT should be used.

ECT should not be used as a sole treatment but should always be part of an overall treatment plan where issues such as losses and the psychological sequelae of traumatic events are appropriately dealt with using psychological therapies. Patients whose depression is understandable in terms of their life experience will usually be treated by psychological methods, but if they are severely ill with their depression so that their safety is threatened, then they should not be deprived of effective treatment just because their depression is understandable. Conversely, patients who show great distress and who may be very unhappy should not be considered candidates for ECT unless they have the symptoms of major depressive illness.

ECT is occasionally indicated for other conditions in those under 18 such as schizophrenia or mania. There are no conditions unique to childhood or adolescence where ECT is indicated.

When should ECT be used?

(1) ECT is hardly ever a first line treatment in childhood or adolescence, although we can envisage situations where this might be so.

> **Case example**
> A 15-year-old girl with a recurrent unipolar depressive illness presents with her fourth episode of major depression. The first episode was at the age of 11. The first and second episodes were treated successfully with a combination of antidepressants, general social support and

regular family interviews. The third major episode at the age of 14 failed to respond to antidepressant drugs or more intensive psychotherapy and the girl made two suicide attempts. She was finally given a course of ECT and responded. She did not wish to take prophylactic medication and relapsed a year later, again with a serious major depression and marked suicidal ideation. In such a case it might be appropriate to consider ECT as a first line treatment.

(2) In general, ECT should be considered after other treatments such as psychotherapy and antidepressant drugs, alone or in combination, have been tried. The indications set out in Chapters 1–3 apply equally to children and adolescents.

Indications for ECT in children aged 12 and under

(1) We have no evidence that ECT is being used in this age group in the UK or Eire.

(2) We do not think there are any clear or definite indications for ECT in this age group.

(3) We would not recommend a ban on ECT in this age group for the reasons set out overleaf.

(4) We realise that the distinction between above 13 and below 13 is an arbitrary one, but we have made it here to emphasise that there is no practice of giving ECT to "children" and no desire to introduce one.

Consent to ECT

(1) Adolescents aged 16–18 are able to consent to and refuse treatment in just the same way as those aged 18 and over. For those under 16 years of age, parental consent is required in England and Wales, but not in Scotland.

(2) In those under 16, even when consent is given by the patient and the parents, we would recommend that an independent second opinion is sought from another child and adolescent psychiatrist. We think that in those under 16 there is sufficient public concern and debate about ECT to make two further opinions desirable clinical practice: one from a child and adolescent psychiatrist and one from another independent psychiatrist from a different clinical unit. We realise that in making this recommendation, we may be seen as helping to perpetuate the view that ECT is a risky or dangerous procedure where special precautions have to be taken, and that this might also be seen as limiting a patient's freedom to choose treatment. On balance, we think that most families would welcome a second opinion and not find it intrusive.

(3) Where consent is not obtained, we recommend that treatment should not be given unless the patient's life is at risk from suicide or physical debilitation secondary to depressive illness.

(4) Where treatment has to be given and where the individual's consent cannot be obtained either because of refusal or incapability to consent, treatment should be given under the relevant legislation (i.e. the Mental Health Act 1983, Mental Health (Scotland) Act 1984 or Mental Health (Northern Ireland) Order 1946). These Acts have no lower age limit.

    (a) Parental consent alone should not be relied on. The Mental Health Act Commission or Mental Welfare Commission in Scotland will automatically be involved. The patient and family have greater protection and access to appeal and second opinion.

    (b) The Act makes specific recommendations about treatment plans.

Should ECT in those under 18 be banned?

(1) If ECT were banned, a small number of individuals would continue to suffer severe distress from their depressive illness and some would die from their depressive illness or suicide. It does not make sense to deprive one segment of the population of a treatment which is the most effective there is for certain psychiatric illnesses.

(2) There is no evidence that ECT is less effective or associated with more adverse effects in those under the age of 18.

(3) We do not think there should be a lower age limit below which ECT is banned, although we think it is extremely unlikely that ECT would ever need to be given to someone under the age of 13. There is an increasing recognition of severe depressive disorders in children of this age and younger. As far as we are aware, no ECT is currently being given to those aged 12 and under in the UK, although again there might be unique clinical circumstances where it might be the best available treatment.

Technical considerations for ECT in those under 18

(1) Seizure threshold decreases with decreasing age. It is particularly important in the young to use an ECT machine that can provide flexible doses of ECT and where stimuli as low as 25 or 50 mCs can be given.

(2) We strongly recommend that seizure threshold is determined at the start of treatment and that initial stimuli should be at the lower end of the range of the ECT machine.

(3) ECT should not be given to those under the age of 18 using a fixed-dose ECT machine. (For details of stimulus dosing see Chapter 22).

(4) Those under 18 requiring ECT are likely to be in-patients. Such patients should be appropriately treated in adolescent psychiatry units rather than adult wards. The ECT session should be arranged so that treatment is given separately from adult wards, although we do not think it is necessary to have separate ECT facilities for those under 18.

How commonly is ECT used in those under 18 years?

(1) A survey of child and adolescent psychiatrists carried out in 1991 by the Child and Adolescent Section of the Royal College of Psychiatrists showed that there were some 65 cases under the age of 18 years treated in the past ten years. Over 60% of these were between 16 and 18 years old. It is likely that this study only detected cases who had been treated by child and adolescent psychiatrists and not adolescents treated in adult wards.

(2) A recent survey in Scotland (Robertson & Freeman, 1995) looked at all ECT clinics (NHS and private). This showed no ECT treatments given to those under 13 years old in the past five years and only six cases given to those under 18 years. As this survey covered all facilities where ECT is given in the country, all those under 18 would be recorded. Translating this to England and Wales, if ECT were being given at the same rate, some 60 cases would have been treated in the past five years.

(3) With such a low rate of treatment, it is very unlikely that any one centre will have more than an occasional experience of treating those under 18. Low numbers also mean that conducting any controlled trials would be impossible. We recommend that a national audit of ECT in those under 18 be carried out, examining all aspects of the ECT process in this group.

Further reading

HARRINGTON, R. (1992) The natural history and treatment of child and adolescent affective disorders. *Journal of Child Psychology and Psychiatry and Allied Disciplines*, **33**, 1287–1302.

PARMAR, R. (1993) Attitudes of child psychiatrists to electroconvulsive therapy. *Psychiatric Bulletin of the Royal College of Psychiatrists*, **17**, 12–13.

POWELL, J. C., SILVEIRA, W. R. & LINDSAY, R. (1988) Pre-pubertal depressive stupor: a case report. *British Journal of Psychiatry*, **153**, 689–692.

ROBERTSON, C. & FREEMAN, C. P. (1995) Scottish survey of ECT clinics. In *Clinical Researh & Audit Group of the Scottish Office Concensus Report on ECT* (ed. C. Freeman). Scotland: CRAG (in press).

7. ECT and obstetrics

T. Lock

ECT in pregnancy

In deciding on the best treatment for an acutely ill pregnant woman, it is important to weigh the likely benefits for the mother against the known risks to the foetus. There have been no controlled trials of somatic treatments in pregnant women, and available literature on the teratogenicity of drug treatments does not allow for firm conclusions about their safety.

Pregnancy is not a contraindication to ECT, or general anaesthesia (Selvin, 1987), and about 350 cases of ECT in pregnancy, including high-risk pregnancies (Wise *et al*, 1984), have been reported. Reluctance to administer ECT to pregnant women may stem from concern about exposing the foetus to potentially harmful hypoxia during seizure activity, and early reports of adverse effects on the foetus associated with Metrazol and insulin seizures. Recent case reports, supported by data obtained by means of sophisticated foetal monitoring techniques, confirm that ECT is not associated with maternal hypoxia or foetal distress when it is administered in the second and third trimesters of pregnancy (Repke & Berger, 1984; Wise *et al*, 1984; Yellowlees & Page, 1990; Varan *et al*, 1985). Foetal heart rate shows a brief response to atropine premedication (tachycardia) and to the tonic phase of the induced seizure (bradycardia), but is otherwise remarkably stable throughout an ECT procedure. Foetal activity remains normal during an ECT treatment, and foetal growth appears to be unaffected by a course of ECT. ECT has not been associated with abnormal uterine contractions or other later complications during pregnancy, labour and delivery, or with complications in postnatal growth and development.

There is a need for detailed reports of successful and unsuccessful case studies, particularly in cases where ECT is administered in the first trimester of pregnancy.

Recommendations

(1) ECT may be prescribed with confidence for pregnant patients in the second and third trimesters of pregnancy:
    (a) where patients display symptom patterns strongly indicative of a good response to ECT;
    (b) when rapid control of symptoms is required;
    (c) where there is an increased risk of toxicity to both mother and foetus when effective dosages of psychotropic drugs are used as an alternative.
(2) Little is known about the effects of ECT in the first trimester of pregnancy.
(3) There is no evidence of a need for routine sophisticated monitoring of maternal and foetal status.
(4) It is advisable to discuss the case with the patient's obstetrician when a psychiatric decision is taken to administer ECT to a pregnant patient.
(5) High-risk pregnancies are not an absolute contraindication to ECT, provided that the patient is jointly managed by a psychiatrist and an obstetrician, and that facilities exist for careful monitoring of maternal and foetal status (Wise *et al*, 1984).

References

REPKE, J. T. & BERGER, N. G. (1984) Electroconvulsive therapy in pregnancy. *Obstetrics and Gynaecology*, **63** (suppl. 3), 39S–41S.

SELVIN, B. L. (1987) Electroconvulsive therapy – 1987. *Anaesthesiology*, **67**, 367–385.
VARAN, L. R., GILLIESON, M. S., SKENE, D. S., *et al* (1985) ECT in an acutely psychotic pregnant woman with actively aggressive (homicidal) impulses. *Canadian Journal of Psychiatry*, **30**, 363–367.
WISE, M. G., WARD, S. C., TOWNSEND-PARCHMAN, W., *et al* (1984) Case report of ECT during high-risk pregnancy. *American Journal of Psychiatry*, **141**, 99–101.
YELLOWLEES, P. M. & PAGE, T. (1990) Safe use of electroconvulsive therapy in pregnancy. *Medical Journal of Australia*, **153**, 679–680.

ECT and postpartum psychosis

Symptomatology in 80% of cases of postpartum psychosis is predominantly affective: 40% present with manic and schizomanic syndromes, 40% with depressed affect and delusions, and 20% with predominantly Type I (florid) schizophrenic symptoms – often with a marked affective component, or symptoms suggestive of an acute organic brain syndrome (Meltzer & Kumar, 1985).

Treatment is essentially the same as for similar conditions not associated with childbirth. In a review of the literature, Brockington *et al* (1982) recommended that ECT should be used if there is no response to alternative treatment within four weeks. There have been no controlled trials comparing the efficacy of ECT with psychotropics in puerperal psychosis, but clinical experience suggests that ECT may be considered the treatment of choice for most psychotic puerperal women with marked affective symptoms. Delusional depression, in particular, indicates a good outcome to treatment (Brandon *et al*, 1984; Oates, 1986). Furthermore, ECT offers rapid control of symptoms and a lower risk of toxicity to a lactating mother and her breast-fed infant than with psychotropic drugs.

References

BRANDON, S., COWLEY, P., MCDONALD, C., *et al* (1984) Electroconvulsive therapy: results in depressive illness from the Leicestershire trial. *British Medical Journal*, **228**, 22–25.
BROCKINGTON, I. F., WINOKUR, G. & DEAN, C. (1982) Puerperal psychosis. In *Motherhood and Mental Illness* (eds I. F. Brockington & R. Kumar), pp. 37–69. London: Academic.
MELTZER, E. S. & KUMAR, R. (1985) Puerperal mental illness, clinical features and classification – a study of 142 mother-and-baby admissions. *British Journal of Psychiatry*, **147**, 647–654.
OATES, M. (1986) The role of electroconvulsive therapy in the treatment of postnatal mental illness. In *Current Approaches to the Treatment of Postnatal Mental Illness*. Southampton: Duphar.

8. ECT in learning disability psychiatry

R. McClelland

Reported prevalence rates for affective psychosis in the learning disabled vary from 1.2–2.8%. No double-blind study testing the efficacy of ECT in this population has yet been reported and descriptions of its efficacy have taken the form of five case reports.

(1) Bates & Smeltzer (1982) described a 21-year-old learning disabled man who had suffered recurrent episodes of self-injurious behaviour from childhood, associated with insomnia and weight loss, and refractory to both intensive behaviour modification programmes and to various psychotropic medications, including lithium. The aberrant behaviour, mainly head-banging, became so severe that it was judged to be life-threatening, and judicial intervention (Ohio State Law) was granted to administer ECT. Following treatment all symptoms resolved but relapse recurred at four months.

(2) Merrill (1990) reported on a profoundly learning disabled woman with a history of at least six episodes of apparent affective illness, characterised by a lack of responsiveness, appetite and participation in activities. There was notable agitation with screaming and crying alternating with hysterical laughter and refusal of food and fluids. Chemotherapy, including major neuroleptics, lithium and a tricyclic antidepressant, was unsuccessful, and judicial approval (Minnesota State Law) was granted to administer ECT. After the sixth treatment all symptoms resolved.

(3) Kearns (1987) described a 67-year-old learning disabled man with Cotard's syndrome. The patient expressed nihilistic ideas and told carers that he had no body and legs, that his bowels were missing, and that as he was dead he believed that he should be in the hospital mortuary. After six ECT treatments the patient returned gradually to his premorbid state.

(4) Warren & Holroyd (1989), in their paper on major depression in Down's syndrome, described five patients with trisomy 21, who had been referred for evaluation of dementia, and were instead found to have major depression. In addition to the more familiar indicators of affective illness such as loss of appetite, weight and sleep, a common theme in these patients' symptomatology was loss of adaptive skills and, in three of the five, incontinence of urine or faeces was reported. All were treated with amitriptyline. Two of the patients recovered fully on this, but the remaining three showed little or no improvement and were treated with ECT which led to a full recovery.

(5) Goldstein & Jensvold (1989) described a 68-year-old man with full scale IQ of 63 and multiple somatic complaints. Complaints persisted despite surgery for an undescended testicle and gallstones over a three year period. Psychotic depression was diagnosed but unsuccessfully treated with courses of trazodone, amitriptyline and imipramine. A course of ten unilateral ECT treatments was administered and his somatic preoccupations rapidly subsided.

The information available would suggest that ECT is a useful therapeutic option for a minority of patients where: (a) the patient's behaviour or symptoms, or both, are suggestive of severe depressive illness; and (b) where adequate trials of chemotherapy have failed. The issue of consent may worry some psychiatrists, and relevant guidance is given in Part III, "Consent to ECT".

References

BATES, W. J. & SMELTZER, D. J. (1982) Electroconvulsive treatment of psychotic self-injurious behaviour in a patient with some mental retardation. *American Journal of Psychiatry,* **139**, 1355–1356.

GOLDSTEIN, M. Z. & JENSVOLD, M. F. (1989) ECT treatment of an elderly mentally retarded man. *Psychosomatics,* **30**, 104–106.

KEARNS, A. (1987) Cotard's syndrome in a mentally handicapped man. *British Journal of Psychiatry,* **150**, 112–114.

MERRILL, R. D. (1990) ECT for a patient with profound mental retardation. *American Journal of Psychiatry,* **147**, 256–257.

WARREN, A. C. & HOLROYD, S. (1989) Major depression in Down's syndrome. *British Journal of Psychiatry,* **155**, 202–205.

9. Safe ECT practice in physically ill patients

S. M. Benbow

This section deals with the use of ECT when certain medical conditions are present. Any concurrent medical conditions and the balance of risks and benefits in individual cases should be considered before making a decision to treat with ECT. Bilateral ECT is the preferred treatment for those people whose medical conditions make it advisable to minimise the number of anaesthetics administered. Caffeine has been used to increase seizure duration in some patients with concurrent medical illnesses who had very short seizures despite maximal device settings (Lurie & Coffey, 1990).

Stroke

ECT has been used successfully and safely in post-stroke depressive illnesses. Alexopoulos *et al* (1984) included in their series a patient who received treatment four days after a cerebral infarction documented by computerised tomography scan. Murray *et al* (1986) reported four people treated with ECT within one month of having strokes.

Most practitioners prefer to avoid the use of ECT within three months of stroke, but recent stroke is not an absolute contraindication.

Dementing illnesses

There have been case reports of successful ECT treatment of people with dementing illnesses, including Alzheimer's disease (Snow & Wells, 1981), normal pressure hydrocephalus (McAllister & Price, 1982), Huntington's chorea (Perry, 1983) and Creuzfeldt-Jakob disease (McAllister & Price, 1982), but they are more likely to develop confusional states. The confusion gradually improves and eventually resolves but may last up to 6–8 weeks (Summers *et al*, 1979; Tsuang *et al*, 1979).

Nelson & Rosenberg (1991) carried out a retrospective analysis of patients over the age of 60 treated with ECT over a four year period. Twenty-one of 103 patients with depression and dementia were treated with ECT (20.4%) and 84 depressed people without concurrent dementias (17.5%) received ECT. The response to ECT did not differ between the two groups, but confusion scores were significantly higher in the dual diagnosis group, and post-ECT confusion score correlated with the degree of dementia.

In treating a patient with a known dementing illness, unilateral ECT may be preferable to minimise cognitive side-effects, but a patient who fails to respond should be changed to bilateral treatment (Abrams, 1992). Careful monitoring of cognitive function during ECT is important, with attention to factors which may help to decrease the severity of any adverse effect, for example, concomitant psychotropic drugs, dose of anaesthetic medication, and stimulus intensity. Many clinicians continue a course of ECT despite confusion, provided other possible causes (for example, infection) have been excluded and treatment factors have been minimised.

Epilepsy and other neurological conditions

Hsiao *et al* (1987) reviewed the use of ECT in neurological conditions. They concluded that diagnosed, treated epilepsy does not present a significant risk factor for ECT if underlying lesions, structural or vascular, are excluded. The stimulus intensity and dose of anticonvulsant drugs may need to be adjusted to ensure an adequate seizure. Patients with spontaneous epilepsy may be predisposed to lengthy seizures which may need to be terminated by an intravenous infusion of general anaesthetic, lidocaine or benzodiazepines. Patients with coexisting pathophysiological states which lower seizure threshold may similarly be predisposed to lengthy seizures.

There are single case reports of the safe use of ECT in a range of neurological conditions, including Friedreich's ataxia (Casey, 1991), following craniotomy for meningioma (Hsiao & Evans, 1984), raised intracranial pressure (Dubovsky *et al*, 1985), mental impairment (Goldstein & Jensvold, 1989; Merrill, 1990), Down's syndrome (Lazarus *et al*, 1990), treated hydrocephalus related to Paget's disease of the skull (Cardno & Simpson, 1991), and chronic subdural haematoma (Malek-Ahmadi *et al*, 1990).

ECT has been used successfully in the presence of intracranial aneurysm (Husum *et al*, 1983), using methods of preventing elevated blood pressure and heart rate during treatment. Post-craniotomy the electrodes should be placed at a distance from the cranial defect. By six months after cerebral trauma there is probably little increased risk from ECT (Hsiao *et al*, 1987). ECT has been used in patients with neurosyphilis (Shapiro & Goldberg, 1957), but active central nervous system infection should be treated first. The use of ECT in neurological conditions appears safe, but space-occupying lesions with increased intracranial pressure, recent cerebral trauma, and active central nervous system infection are of special concern. The underlying disorder should be fully assessed and, wherever possible, treated first.

Cardiovascular disease

People with known cardiac disease have an increased rate of cardiac complications during ECT (Gerring & Shields, 1982; Alexopoulos *et al*, 1984), particularly older patients (Cattan *et al*, 1990) and those with a higher risk status using the American Society of Anaesthesiologists (ASA) classification system (Burke *et al*, 1985). Age and ASA rating correlated, suggesting that the increasing health problems of older people increase their risk. Nevertheless, ECT has been used safely in people with dissecting aortic aneurysm (Rosenfeld *et al*, 1988; Devanand *et al*, 1990), in those on anticoagulant treatment (Loo *et al*, 1985) and in people with implanted cardiac pacemakers (Regestein & Lind, 1980; Alexopoulos *et al*, 1984).

Precautions are advisable in people with known cardiovascular disease, and the cardiovascular status of elderly people should be assessed before ECT. At-risk individuals should be evaluated by a cardiologist or other experienced physician. Electrocardiogram monitoring may be advisable before, during and for a minimum of 15 minutes after each treatment. Staff trained in cardio-pulmonary resuscitation and the emergency treatment of arrhythmias should be available. In high-risk individuals it may be necessary to administer ECT in a cardiac care unit with specialist staff at hand. Manesksha (1991) has reviewed techniques used to modify the cardiovascular response in at-risk patients. In patients with aortic homografts, a history of aortic dissection or concurrent untreated aortic aneurysm, extensive precautions may sometimes be necessary to prevent or minimise post-ECT elevations in blood pressure and heart rate. Full muscular relaxation is important in people with abdominal aortic aneurysm (Goumeniouk *et al*, 1990). Pacemakers should be checked for breaks in wires or faulty insulation, and during treatment the patient and the monitoring equipment should be completely insulated from the ground (Abrams, 1992). Following myocardial infarction, ECT should be delayed for as long as possible and is probably safer after three months (Perrin, 1961). Since these patients may need anti-arrhythmic and anti-hypertensive drugs, and the administration of 100% oxygen by positive pressure before, during and after the seizure, specialist advice should be sought (Abrams, 1992).

Other medical conditions

In the presence of severe unstable cervical spine disease, ECT has been used with maximal muscle relaxation and minimal neck manipulation (Kellner *et al*, 1991).

Recommendations

If physically ill people need ECT:

(1) there are no absolute contraindications.
(2) all coexisting medical conditions should be assessed and, where possible, treated before ECT.
(3) the balance between risks and benefits must always be weighed.
(4) as far as possible, patients and their families should be involved in discussions about the treatment, its risks and benefits.
(5) ECT is not a treatment in itself for any of the above conditions (with the exception of epilepsy: see Chapter 4).

References

ABRAMS, R. (1992) The medical physiology of ECT. In *Electroconvulsive Therapy* (ed. R. Abrams), pp. 47–76. Oxford: Oxford University Press.

ALEXOPOULOS, G. S., SHAMOIAN, C. J., LUCAS, J., *et al* (1984) Medical problems of geriatric psychiatric patients and younger controls during electroconvulsive therapy. *Journal of the American Geriatrics Society*, **32**, 651–654.

BURKE, W. J., RUTHERFORD, J. L., ZORUMSKI, C. F., *et al* (1985) Electroconvulsive therapy and the elderly. *Comprehensive Psychiatry*, **26**, 480–486.

CARDNO, A. G. & SIMPSON, C. J. (1991) Electroconvulsive therapy in Paget's disease and hydrocephalus. *Convulsive Therapy*, **7**, 48-51.

CASEY, D. A. (1991) Electroconvulsive therapy and Friedreich's ataxia. *Convulsive Therapy*, **7**, 45–47.

CATTAN, R. A., BARRY, P. P., MEAD, G., *et al* (1990) Electroconvulsive therapy in octogenarians. *Journal of the American Geriatrics Society*, **38**, 753–758.

DEVANAND, D. P., MALITZ, S. & SACKEIM, H. A. (1990) ECT in a patient with aortic aneurysm. *Journal of Clinical Psychiatry*, **51**, 255–256.

DUBOVSKY, S. L., GAY, M., FRANKS, R. D., *et al* (1985) ECT in the presence of increased intracranial pressure and respiratory failure – case report. *Journal of Clinical Psychiatry*, **46**, 489–491.

GERRING, J. P. & SHIELDS, H. M. (1982) The identification and management of patients with a high risk for cardiac arrythmias during modified ECT. *Journal of Clinical Psychiatry*, **43**, 140–143.

GOLDSTEIN, M. Z. & JENSVOLD, M. F. (1989) ECT treatment of an elderly mentally retarded man. *Psychosomatics*, **30**, 104–106.

GOUMENIOUK, A. D., FRY, P. D. & ZIS, A. P. (1990) Abdominal aortic aneurysm and ECT administration. *Convulsive Therapy*, **6**, 55–57.

HSIAO, J. K. & EVANS, D. L. (1984) ECT in a depressed patient after craniotomy. *American Journal of Psychiatry*, **141**, 442–444.

——, MESSENHEIMER, J. A. & EVANS, D. L. (1987) ECT and neurological disorders. *Convulsive Therapy*, **3**, 121–136.

HUSUM, B., VESTER-ANDERSEN, T., BUCHMANN, G., *et al* (1983) Electroconvulsive therapy and intra-cranial aneurysm. *Anaesthesia*, **38**, 1205–1207.

KELLNER, C. H., TOLHURST, J. E. & BURNS, C. M. (1991) ECT in the presence of severe cervical spine disease. *Convulsive Therapy*, **7**, 52–55.

LAZARUS, A., JAFFE, R. L. & DUBIN, W. R. (1990) Electroconvulsive therapy and major depression in Down's syndrome. *Journal of Clinical Psychiatry*, **51**, 422–425.

LOO, H., CUCHE, H. & BENKELFAT, C. (1985) Electroconvulsive therapy during anticoagulant therapy. *Convulsive Therapy*, **1**, 258–262.

LURIE, S. N. & COFFEY, C. E. (1990) Caffeine-modified electroconvulsive therapy in depressed patients with medical illness. *Journal of Clinical Psychiatry*, **51**, 154–157.

MALEK-AHMADI, P., BECEIRO, J. R., MCNEIL, B. W., *et al* (1990) Electroconvulsive therapy and chronic subdural haematoma. *Convulsive Therapy*, **6**, 38–41.

MANEKSHA, F. R. (1991) Hypertension and tachycardia during electroconvulsive therapy – to treat or not to treat? *Convulsive Therapy*, **7**, 28–35.

McAllister, T. W. & Price, T. R. P. (1982) Severe depressive pseudodementia with and without dementia. *American Journal of Psychiatry,* **139**, 626–629.

Merrill, R. D. (1990) ECT for a patient with profound mental retardation. *American Journal of Psychiatry,* **147**, 256–257.

Murray, G. B., Shea, V. & Conn, D. K. (1986) Electroconvulsive therapy for post-stroke depression. *Journal of Clinical Psychiatry,* **47**, 258–260.

Nelson, J. P. & Rosenberg, D. R. (1991) ECT treatment of demented elderly patients with major depression – A retrospective study of efficacy and safety. *Convulsive Therapy,* **7**, 157–165.

Perrin, G. M. (1961) Cardiovascular aspects of electric shock therapy. *Acta Psychiatrica Scandinavica,* **36**, 1–45.

Perry, G. F. (1983) ECT for dementia and catatonia. *Journal of Clinical Psychiatry,* **44**, 117.

Regestein, Q. R. & Lind, L. J. (1980) Management of electroconvulsive treatment of an elderly woman with severe hypertension and cardiac arrhythmias. *Comprehensive Psychiatry,* **21**, 288–291.

Rosenfeld, J. E., Glassberg, S. & Sherrid, M. (1988) Administration of ECT four years after aortic aneurysm dissection. *American Journal of Psychiatry,* **145**, 128–129.

Shapiro, M. F. & Goldberg, H. H. (1957) Electroconvulsive therapy in patients with structural disease of the central nervous system. *American Journal of Medical Science,* **233**, 186–195.

Snow, S. S. & Wells, C. E. (1981) Case studies in neuropsychiatry – diagnosis and treatment of co-existent dementia and depression. *Journal of Clinical Psychiatry,* **42**, 439–441.

Summers, W. K., Robins, E. & Reich, T. (1979) The natural history of acute organic mental syndrome after bilateral electroconvulsive therapy. *Biological Psychiatry,* **14**, 905–912.

Tsuang, M. T., Tidball, J. S. & Geller, D. (1979) ECT in a depressed patient with shunt in place for normal pressure hydrocephalus. *American Journal of Psychiatry,* **136**, 1205–1206.

10. ECT, violence and other offending behaviour

P. Taylor

There is no case for prescribing ECT to alleviate violent or offending behaviour *per se*. For a few patients who are suffering from a psychotic illness which has not quickly responded to antipsychotic medication, and where antisocial acts arise directly from psychosis, ECT may limit the acts by alleviating this.

The most common link between antisocial behaviour and psychosis is between violence and schizophrenia with a predominantly delusional presentation (Taylor *et al*, in press), although to a much lesser extent those with affective psychosis and delusions may also pose a risk. Only one study seems to have made explicit a possible specific advantage for ECT for those with violent propensities. Smith *et al* (1967) noted that among people with schizophrenia the problems that responded most significantly and favourably to an ECT/chlorpromazine combination rather than chlorpromazine alone were hostility (not violence) and ideas of persecution. Taken together, the most recent studies of ECT for schizophrenia, including double-blind approaches, suggest that ECT may speed up the response to anti-psychotic medication, particularly in respect of the most classically schizophrenic symptomatology (Taylor, 1990). There seems little justification in giving ECT as a treatment in isolation, although, especially in forensic psychiatric practice, occasional patients tolerate neuroleptic medication very poorly. For people with chronic, intractable symptomatology, with or without accompanying violence, the evidence is against any specific benefit from ECT.

References

SMITH, K., SURPHLIS, W. R. P., GYNTHER, M. D., *et al* (1967) ECT–chlorpromazine and chlorpromazine compared in the treatment of schizophrenia. *Journal of Nervous and Mental Disease,* **144**, 284–290.

TAYLOR, P. J. (1990) Schizophrenia and ECT – a case for a change in prescription? In *Dilemmas and Difficulties in the Management of Psychiatric Patients* (eds K. Hawton & P. Cowan). Oxford: Oxford University Press.

——, MULLEN, P. & WESSELY, S. (1995) Psychosis, violence and crime. In *Forensic Psychiatry – Clinical, Legal and Ethical Issues* (eds J. Gunn & P. J. Taylor). Oxford: Heinemann-Butterworth (in press).

11. Non-convulsive electric shock treatment
T. Lock

Placebo ECT and sham ECT

The term *placebo* generally refers to inert or harmless substances or treatments that nevertheless may exert powerful or even specific therapeutic effects because of the patient's belief in them. It is inaccurate to describe an ECT procedure from which the electrical shock (and/or induced convulsion) is omitted as 'placebo ECT', for the induction of general anaesthesia and muscle relaxation by means of the administration of two and perhaps three powerful drugs is not a placebo intervention: The terms 'sham' or 'fake' ECT should be used.

It is essential that patients give real consent to their treatment (see Part III). In clinical trials where sham ECT has been given, the consent form has included a statement indicating that the patient might receive either 'real' or 'partial' (i.e. sham or fake) ECT. The surprising finding from the half-dozen studies in the literature where real and sham ECT have been compared is that sham ECT is clearly a powerful antidepressant treatment although not as powerful as real ECT. It would certainly be possible from these findings to make a case for the clinical efficacy of repeated anaesthesia for patients with depressive illness. In these studies, however, the patient knew that there was a chance that they might receive some or all their treatment as real ECT. We are not aware of any studies that have demonstrated the efficacy of repeated anaesthesia where the patient was certain that general anaesthesia was the only treatment they were getting. Consent to what the patient believes to be real ECT is not valid if sham ECT is then intentionally administered instead.

Recommendations

(1) It is misleading to refer to sham ECT as placebo ECT with the implication that this is a risk-free and harmless procedure.
(2) Patients should not be deceived about the nature, purpose or likely consequences of ECT, however well meaning this deception may be.
(3) It is the view of the Special Committee on ECT that sham ECT is not a reasonable or ethical treatment, and we cannot envisage any circumstances where it is reasonable to give sham ECT in the course of routine clinical practice.

Dose titration: subconvulsive stimulations

The aim of dose titration is to determine the minimum amount of electrical stimulation which induces a seizure by a process of repeated stimulations using progressively higher stimulus doses (see "Stimulus dosing"). This may entail administering one or more sub-convulsive ECT treatments. The sub-convulsive stimulations have no therapeutic benefit other than alerting the operator to the fact that the stimulus dose used is below the patient's seizure threshold.

Recommendation

If two stimulations have failed to induce an adequate seizure (i.e. a seizure which is likely to have a therapeutic effect), stimulus dosing policies should attempt to ensure that the third stimulation induces an adequate seizure. This may necessitate a relatively large increase in the amount of the stimulus so as to increase the likelihood of it being above the patient's seizure threshold. If this is encountered during the process of seizure threshold titration, determination of seizure threshold could be completed at the next treatment session.

Aversive shock treatment

Aversive shock treatment has nothing in common with ECT, other than both entail an electrical stimulation. The aim of ECT is to induce a convulsion. With aversive shock treatment, the aim is to administer a painful (or 'noxious') non-convulsive electric shock in clear consciousness. Aversive shock treatment was a behaviourist technique based on conditional learning theory, and the purpose of the technique is to bring about a change of behaviour. The technique has been used fairly widely in learning experiments involving laboratory animals – in which case it is not being used therapeutically – but it has also been used in a therapeutic sense in the treatment of conditions characterised by maladaptive behaviour (e.g. certain types of sexual deviancy). Nowadays aversive shock treatment is rarely used and many regard its use as unethical.

It is important to recognise that some members of the public have a preconceived belief that ECT is a form of punishment, and this may be a reason for refusing to consent to ECT. In some cases, this belief is based on powerful negative images, such as the use of punishing electric shocks in the film "One Flew over the Cuckoo's Nest".

Ectron Ectonustim machines (see Appendix VI) have a 'cerebral stimulator' which delivers a weak non-convulsive stimulus. One of the two uses for this function recommended by the manufacturer is to give a painful stimulus in conjunction with therapeutic suggestions for the treatment of hysteria. This amounts to aversive shock therapy.

Recommendations

(1) It is sometimes necessary to reassure patients and their relatives that contemporary ECT is in no way punitive.

(2) ECT has nothing in common with aversive shock therapy, and it is the view of the ECT Committee that the administration of painful sub-convulsive electrical stimuli is not a reasonable or ethical treatment in contemporary psychiatric practice.

12. ECT and other conditions
T. Lock & R. McClelland

Diabetes mellitus

Recent interest in the effects of ECT in diabetes mellitus can be traced to Fakhri's (1966) report of the normalisation of fasting blood sugar in a 50-year-old man with diabetes mellitus who received ECT for depression. Fakhri *et al* (1980) confirmed these findings in a series of 14 patients with non-insulin dependent diabetes.

The interpretation of these findings has been challenged by more recent investigations of depression, diabetes and ECT. Insulin-dependent diabetes mellitus is reported to be more difficult to control when patients are chronically depressed (Crammer & Gillies, 1981; Kronfol *et al*, 1981), and contrary evidence exists that ECT appears to have a diabetogenic effect in insulin dependent diabetics (Yudofsky & Rosenthal, 1980; Finestone & Weiner, 1984). It has been suggested that, in the case of Fakhri's non-insulin dependent patients, the hyperglycaemia which responded to ECT was, in fact, secondary to endogenous changes in cortical steroids associated with their depressive state (Jenike, 1982).

Recommendation

Earlier evidence that ECT has a therapeutic effect in diabetes mellitus has not been substantiated, and ECT is not recommended as a specific treatment for diabetes mellitus.

References

CRAMMER, J. & GILLIES, C. (1981) Psychiatric aspects of diabetes mellitus: diabetes and depression. *British Journal of Psychiatry*, **139**, 171–172.
FAKHRI, O. (1966) Blood sugar after electroplexy. *Lancet, ii*, 587.
——, FADHLI, A. A. & EL RAWDI, R. M. (1980) Effective electroconvulsive therapy on diabetes mellitus. *Lancet, ii*, 775–777.
FINESTONE, D. H. & WEINER, R. D. (1984) Effects of ECT on diabetes mellitus. *Acta Neurologica Scandinavica*, **70**, 321–326.
JENIKE, M. A. (1982) ECT and diabetes mellitus. *American Journal of Psychiatry*, **139**, 136.
KRONFOL, Z., GREDEN, J. & CARROLL, B. (1981) Psychiatric aspects of diabetes mellitus – diabetes and depression. *British Journal of Psychiatry*, **139**, 172.
YUDOFSKY, S. C. & ROSENTHAL, N. E. (1980) ECT in a depressed patient with adult onset diabetes mellitus. *American Journal of Psychiatry*, **137**, 100–101.

Obsessive–compulsive disorders

About 90% of patients with obsessive–compulsive disorder (OCD) can be helped by sequential or concurrent drug and behavioural treatment, the effectiveness of which has been demonstrated in clinical trials. Few patients are ever completely 'cured' of their symptoms. There have been no controlled trials of ECT in OCD, but in one large open study ECT was shown to have no therapeutic benefit in the treatment of patients with OCD (Grimshaw, 1965).

Psychic ruminations and/or compulsive behaviours are prevalent in up to 20% of patients presenting with depressive illness (Hamilton, 1989). Patients with established OCD may decompensate for a variety of reasons and develop depressive illness for which ECT may be appropriate.

Recommendations

(1) ECT is unlikely to be effective in the treatment of OCD *per se*.
(2) Failure of drug and behavioural treatment is not an indication for ECT.
(3) ECT may be of benefit to some patients with both obsessive–compulsive and depressive symptoms, particularly when associated with 'endogenous' features and mood-congruent delusions or overvalued ideas.

References

GRIMSHAW, L. (1965) The outcome of obsessive compulsive disorder – a follow-up study of 100 cases. *British Journal of Psychiatry*, **111**, 1051–1056.

HAMILTON, M. (1989) Frequency of symptoms in melancholia (depressive illness). *British Journal of Psychiatry*, **154**, 201–206.

Part II. Administration of ECT

13. The ECT suite

C. P. Freeman & J. Lambourn

An area designated as a centre for ECT should exist within each general psychiatry facility. Such a provision is recommended in terms of patient safety and economy of staffing. The priority for such a provision will depend on the number of patients referred for treatment. The minimum requirement for a treatment centre is three rooms. An ideal suite would have five areas, including an ECT office and a final post-ECT waiting area.

The waiting area should be comfortable and informally equipped. Patients dislike the waiting period and their attendance at the centre should be booked to provide a smooth throughput with a minimum of waiting. The size of this room should not, therefore, be calculated for the number of patients attending for each treatment session, but with the aim of providing a relaxing environment of about 20–40 square metres with distractions, for example, an outside window, fish tank, pictures and magazines. Leading off this room should be toilet facilities.

Accessible from the waiting area should be a treatment room of approximately 10 square metres where the patient is assisted onto a trolley and receives treatment. (The practice of patients mounting trolleys in an intermediate room and waiting again before being pushed into the treatment area is to be deprecated, as it produces increasing patient anxiety.) This room requires good, but not harsh illumination and ventilation. Provision for positive pressure respiration with oxygen, suction and emergency resuscitation are mandatory. A work surface and sink with hot and cold water are necessary.

There should be good sound-proofing between the waiting area and treatment room, and waiting patients should not be exposed to a full view of the treatment room each time the door is opened.

Some form of doorway capable of admitting a trolley is necessary into the recovery area. The trolleys should comfortably accommodate a reclining adult, but be tippable into a head-down position in case of emergency. The wheels should be braked and the provision of collapsible safety side-rails is highly desirable.

A system must be established for calling the anaesthetist from the treatment room to the recovery area in case of emergency. Patients remain in the primary recovery area until they are able to walk and are reorientated. This time will vary with their pretreatment condition and the amount of stimulus they receive. For elderly patients, up to 30 minutes should be allowed. With a throughput of one every five minutes, provision for up to six patients lying on trolleys must be made, plus ample space to manoeuvre these trolleys in an emergency – a minimum provision of 28 square metres.

From the recovery area the patients may be escorted to a final stage area, where delays in transport can necessitate the whole of a unit's patient throughput being accommodated. As in the case of the waiting area, an attempt should be made to provide a relaxed friendly atmosphere, and to that end refreshments are most welcome.

A separate office is required for the administration of the unit. This cannot satisfactorily be carried out from any of the other rooms as patients are bound to be discussed on the telephone, and confidentiality would be broken.

In-patients will be escorted to the unit by a member of the ward nursing staff who should stay with them, attentive to their needs at all times. (Out-patients will have reported to the ward first and have been allocated a supportive nurse.)

Recent trends

Following the introduction of the recent NHS reforms, a trend has emerged – in England at least – for two or more psychiatric facilities to share a common ECT suite, or even for one trust to seek to purchase an ECT service from another. This trend has been driven primarily by economic considerations. There are potential advantages and practical disadvantages inherent in this approach.

Disadvantages

The obvious disadvantage is the need for a group (or groups) of patients to commute, by hospital transport or even private taxi, to and from their base unit and the unit in which the ECT suite is situated. Commuting is not without precedent, as this is what out-patients receiving ECT do. A regular group of commuting patients, however, poses clinical problems.

(1) Patient safety must be ensured while in transit. The need for *individual* escorts must be stressed.
(2) It may not be advisable to transport some elderly, frail or physically ill patients, and it may be more appropriate to admit these patients to the hospital in which the ECT clinic is situated.
(3) It is most definitely not advisable to transport patients who have not recovered adequately from their ECT treatment. As a general rule, it is probably advisable for the commuting patients to be treated at the start of an ECT treatment session so that their recovery can be adequately monitored by ECT clinic staff.

Commuters also pose legal dilemmas, for example, whether or not Mental Health Act papers need to be transferred in cases where the patient and the ECT clinic fall under the management of different trusts. As yet there are no guidelines addressing this issue. One legal issue relates to liability in the event of an accident while patients are in transit.

Advantages

The main advantage of a shared ECT clinic is that resources and staff expertise can be focused on one well used, well staffed and well equipped clinic, rather than continuing to maintain two or more underused, understaffed and inadequately equipped clinics. The consultant in charge of the ECT clinic should, however, ensure that the clinic is not placed in a position whereby existing staffing levels and equipment are expected to cope with an additional influx of commuting patients.

Staffing

Nurses

It must be borne in mind that when an ECT unit is functioning normally, the staff requirements are light, but in the case of an emergency, one must make provision for three unconscious patients, of whom two might not be breathing spontaneously. The minimum requirement of nurses must, therefore, be:

> Waiting room – 1 untrained
> Treatment room – 1 trained plus 1 untrained
> Primary recovery – 1 trained plus 1 untrained
> Post-ECT waiting area – 1 untrained

Medical

> Anaesthetist
> Operating department assistant
> Psychiatrist

14. Equipment for the ECT suite
G. Fergusson

Routine ECT

ECT machine and backup:
> Brief pulse, constant current, with wide output range (see section on ECT machines)
> Appropriate electrodes and conducting gel or solution
> **Note**: an existing machine would suffice as a backup machine in clinics which have purchased an "on-site" maintenance and repair service from certain manufacturers

Trolley or bed with firm base:
> With tilting facility and cot sides, one per patient, until recovery

Oxygen:
> Source delivered by IPPV from either cylinder with reserve or anaesthetic machine and appropriate circuits for supply and scavenging
> One face mask per patient

Suction:
> Plus backup and catheters

Sundries:
> Disposable gloves, mouth gags, airways, syringes, needles, IV cannulae, tape, swabs, skin cleanser/ degreaser

Disposal:
> Safe disposal for sharps and clinical waste

Foot stool:
> Must not have wheels (safety regulations)

Routine monitoring equipment

Log book:
> For patients receiving ECT

For seizure length:
> Either automatic or manual recording of seizure length with stopwatch or clock with a second hand sphygmomanometer for 'Hamilton cuff' method

For BP:
> Manual or automatic sphygmomanometer

Pulse oximeter:
> For oxygen saturation

Capnograph:
> For end tidal carbon dioxide saturation

ECG monitor:
> With electrodes

For machines with built-in EEG monitoring:
> Disposable EEG electrodes (paediatric ECG electrodes are suitable)

Recovery room

Oxygen:
> Source as above

Suction:
> Plus back-up

Monitoring equipment:
> For temperature, pulse and blood pressure

Emergency drugs and equipment:
> Must be easily available

Emergency equipment

Drugs:
  See separate list
Defibrillator:
  With appropriate pads or gel
Laryngoscope:
  Plus backup
Airways maintenance:
  ET tubes and/or laryngeal masks and associated equipment
  Chest drain
IV infusion sets:
  Fluids, stand and associated sundries
  IVP line
Dextrostix:
  Or similar for measurement of blood glucose
Ice packs
Stethoscope
Thermometer
Scissors

Maintenance

An agreement should be in place for maintenance of all equipment either with the manufacturer or the medical physics department

List of drugs

Routine ECT

Anaesthetic induction agent:
  Methohexitone sodium and alternatives
Muscle relaxant:
  Suxamethonium and alternative
Oxygen
Others:
  May include
  (i)   glycopyrronium bromide
  (ii) caffeine
  (iii) midazolam (see below)

Emergency use

First line cardiac arrest tray:
  Adrenaline; 1:10 000 in 10 ml × 2
  Atropine; total dose 3 mg
  Calcium chloride; 1 gm in 10 ml × 2
  Lignocaine; 100 mg in 5 ml × 2
Emergency box including:
  (for anaphylaxis)
  Adrenaline; 1 in 1000
  Hydrocortisone; 500 mg in 4 ml
Antihistamine:
  For example, promethazine; 25 mg in 1 ml
Bronchodilators:
  For example, aminophylline, salbutamol, terbutaline

Cardiovascular stimulants and stabilisers:
>   Adenocur
>   Atropine; 0.5 mg in 1 ml
>   Calcium gluconate; 10% in 10 ml
>   Digoxin
>   Disopyramide, verapamil, nitrates
>   Labetolol, esmolol or propranolol
>   Lignocaine
>   Noradrenaline, isoprenaline or dopamine

Dantrolene:
>   plus sterile water

Diazepam:
>   as Diazemuls; 10 mg in 2 ml

Medazolam (i.v.):
>   10mg in 2 ml (for rapid control of severe post-treatment agitation)

Diuretic:
>   for example, frusemide; 50 mg in 5 ml

IVI:
>   Dextrose; 50% in 25 ml
>   Sodium chloride; 0.9% in a 500 ml bag
>   Sodium bicarbonate; 8.4%, 50 ml (minijet)
>   Sodium bicarbonate; 8.4%, 200 ml (bag)

Naloxone:
>   0.4 mg in 1 ml

Physostigmine or neostigmine

15. Anaesthesia for ECT

K. H. Simpson

Anaesthesia for ECT requires special skill and experience. It should not be given by the same person who also administers ECT, but by an anaesthetist competent to deal with any of its complications in a department which may be away from the main hospital (Selvin, 1987).

The involvement of consultants in anaesthesia for ECT improves the quality of care for patients, facilitates staff training and strengthens the relationship between the departments of anaesthesia and psychiatry (Rich & Smith, 1981; Pippard, 1992).

Each anaesthetic department should have a policy, which all staff should be aware of, on the experience needed before giving unsupervised anaesthesia for ECT. One year of anaesthetic experience and specific instruction by a consultant anaesthetist with an interest in ECT is probably the minimum requirement.

A minimum number of trained staff must be present for a treatment session to take place. As well as the anaesthetist and psychiatrist there must be one person to help wih the anaesthesia and one person to recover *each* patient who has not regained conciousness.

Continuity of care by the anaesthetist is as important as by the psychiatrist involved in giving ECT. As far as possible, rotas of anaesthetists attending only occasionally should be avoided, so that patients are regularly anaesthetised by as few doctors as is practicable and the anaesthesia can be individually tailored, assisted by careful recording of anaesthetic regimens and the patient's responses to each treatment. These should include anaesthetic drugs, doses, nature of ventilation, cardiorespiratory changes, seizure quality and duration, time to recovery and postoperative problems.

Good communications must be maintained between anaesthetist, psychiatrist and nurses in the ward and clinic. The anaesthetist should be given concise written information about each patient and their status under the Mental Health Act 1983.

Assessment of patients before ECT

A detailed medical history and a full physical examination are necessary.

(1) Cardiovascular problems are important, as profound haemodynamic changes accompany ECT.
(2) Anaesthesia may be hazardous in patients with serious chest disease.
(3) Bad or loose dentition should be noted, as inhalation of broken or dislodged teeth may occur during treatment or recovery.
(4) Gross obesity or hiatus hernia bring an increased risk of aspiration of gastric contents.
(5) Some muscular and neurological disorders make anaesthesia difficult (see contraindications).
(6) Arthritis in the jaws and neck may cause airway problems.
(7) Enquiries should be made about current medication, drug allergies and pregnancy, and about previous anaesthesia: possible problems include anaphylaxis, emesis, delayed recovery, suxamethonium apnoea, porphyria and susceptibility to malignant hyperthermia.

Investigations

It is important not to add to the discomfort of patients awaiting ECT by unnecessary investigations, but all patients should have a full blood count.

(1) Afro-Carribean, Middle Eastern, Asian and Eastern Mediterranean patients must be sickle-cell tested.

(2) Serum urea and electrolytes should be measured in patients on diuretics or lithium and in those suffering from dehydration, renal, cardiac or liver disease.

(3) All patients should have their urine tested for the presence of blood, glucose or protein.

(4) Blood sugar should be measured using a finger prick prior to anaesthesia in all diabetics.

(5) A chest X-ray is only needed if there are symptoms or signs of cardiorespiratory disease.

(6) An electrocardiogram (ECG) is needed in patients with symptoms or signs of cardiovascular disease, including hypertension.

(7) Wherever possible any physical illness should be controlled before ECT is given; in particular, diabetics should be stabilised, dehydration corrected (it diminishes the efficacy of ECT) and anaemia, thyroid or adrenal disorder dealt with.

(8) Nevertheless, the anaesthetist must remember that treatment with antidepressants has a mortality and so has severe depressive illness. Anaesthesia should be refused only after careful consideration and consultation, usually by senior staff.

(9) If unfit patients cannot be treated in the ECT unit, it may sometimes be possible to anaesthetise them in the main operating theatres, which may have better monitoring and resuscitation facilities.

Contraindications to anaesthesia for ECT

There are probably few absolute contraindications but many cases in which the balance of risks and benefit must be carefully weighed.

(1) Old age alone is insufficient reason to refuse treatment (Malcolm & Peet, 1989).

(2) The desirability of ECT in the presence of uncontrolled hypertension, severe myocardial ischaemia, stenotic valvular disease or aortic aneurysm should be carefully considered. It should be avoided in patients with phaeochromocytoma.

(3) Patients with cardiac pacemakers can safely receive ECT as virtually no ECT current passes through the heart; the patient should be isolated from the ground and the ECG should be monitored during treatment and recovery.

(4) Thrombophlebitis is a contraindication to ECT because of the risk of embolisation, but treatment may be given once the patient is anticoagulated.

(5) ECT should be deferred where possible in patients who have had a myocardial infarction within the preceding three months, and those with untreated heart block or cardiac failure should be deferred until after treatment has been instigated.

(6) Anaesthesia should be deferred in patients with an upper respiratory tract infection.

(7) Most patients with chronic airways disease can be treated if their respiratory function is optimised.

(8) Upper airway obstruction due to arthritis, dental abscess, facial deformity, tumour or laryngeal disease precludes treatment.

(9) Patients with myopathy, myasthenia gravis, muscular dystrophy and susceptibility to malignant hyperthermia should not be anaesthetised in a department remote from a main general hospital. Severe muscle spasm or muscle weakness may occur during anaesthesia or recovery; however, there have been no reports of malignant hyperthermia being triggered during ECT (Johnson & Santos, 1983).

(10) A patient who has suffered a cerebrovascular accident within three months or who has an untreated intracranial aneurysm should not receive ECT if it can be avoided.

(11) It is possible to treat patients with cerebral tumours (Maltbie *et al*, 1980), but with raised intracranial pressure it is especially hazardous.

(12) Acute closed angle glaucoma is a contraindication to ECT, as intraocular pressure increases during treatment may damage the eye.

(13) The desirability of ECT should be carefully considered if the patient is pregnant, but the indications are that ECT can be given safely (Selvin, 1987).

(14) Patients with a haemoglobin concentration of less than 10 g/dl should not usually receive elective anaesthesia until the anaemia is corrected.

(15) Patients with sickle-cell trait can be treated safely, but those with sickle-cell disease may develop an acute crisis and it is not appropriate to anaesthetise them in the ECT unit.

(16) Patients with severe metabolic problems, for example, hepatorenal disease, should not be treated in a remote department.

Preparation for ECT

(1) The most important aspect of preparation of patients is good liaison between the anaesthetist and the ward staff.

(2) A drug history should be taken, since many drugs alter seizure threshold and may alter the efficacy of ECT.

(3) Patients on tricyclic antidepressants are more likely to develop cardiac arrhythmias, but may also be protected against vagal stimulation.

(4) Benzodiazepines reduce seizure intensity and duration.

(5) Patients on membrane stabilising drugs, such as anticonvulsants or beta blockers, may have a modified response to ECT.

(6) Caffeine may augment seizure duration and the efficacy of treatment.

(7) Oral hypoglycaemics should be withheld on the morning of treatment because of the risk of hypoglycaemia. They can be safely given once the patient has recovered from the anaesthetic and had a drink.

(8) Medication for intercurrent medical conditions should be continued because of the risk of hypoglycaemia. The routine discontinuation of monoamine oxidase inhibitors prior to anaesthesia has been questioned (El Ganzouri *et al*, 1985) and is not now thought to be necessary.

(9) Diabetic patients should have their blood glucose concentration measured and normal diabetic management should be resumed as soon after ECT as possible.

(10) All patients should be starved for at least six hours before treatment.

(11) Heavy meals late in the evening prior to ECT should be avoided, especially in patients taking antidepressant medication which slows gastric emptying.

(12) Obese patients or those with oesophageal reflux should receive H_2 blockers and non-particulate antacids prior to anaesthesia.

Premedication

(1) Sedative premedication is undesirable as it may decrease seizure duration and prolong recovery. It was suggested that deaths due to ECT were related to vagal bradycardia and could be prevented by routine atropinization (Bankhead *et al*, 1950). However, deaths were related to hypoxaemia rather than vagal overactivity. Atropine does not contribute to cardiac stability or produce consistent drying of secretions (Wyant & Macdonald, 1980), and injections producing a dry mouth and blurred vision are unnecessary. Subcutaneous or intramuscular atropine before ECT should be avoided.

(2) As well as causing discomfort, atropine predisposes patients to cardiac arrhythmias and should be avoided in most patients, except for the specific management of bradycardia.

(3) If an antisialogogue is needed, glycopyrrolate produces comparable antisialogogue activity to atropine but has less effect on heart rate (Greenan *et al*, 1983).

(4) All anticholinergic drugs reduce lower oesophageal sphincter tone and may predispose to regurgitation of gastric contents.

Anaesthetic induction agents

(1)   Gaseous induction of anaesthesia is best avoided in most patients requiring ECT, as it is slow and may be frightening.

(2)   Anaesthesia is usually induced using intravenous drugs, and it has to be accepted that these will all reduce seizure duration compared with unmodified ECT (Ayd, 1961).

(3)   Methohexitone is the agent of choice, in a dose of 0.75–0.9 mg/kg. Higher doses decrease seizure duration and increase postictal amnesia (Miller *et al*, 1985).

(4)   Methohexitone can be a painful injection and 10 mg of lignocaine can be added to reduce discomfort; the addition of this small dose of lignocaine does not reduce seizure activity (Simpson *et al*, 1989), but is seldom necessary. The use of a larger vein may reduce pain on injection, but veins in the antecubital fossa should be avoided because of the risk of intra-arterial injection.

(5)   Thiopentone increases cardiac arrhythmias 2–4 fold compared with methohexitone (Woodruff *et al*, 1968). Seizure duration and the number of ECT treatments required are similar after the two drugs (Strömgren *et al*, 1980). Thiopentone was reported to prolong recovery compared with methohexitone (Pitts *et al*, 1968), but a later study showed that the time to return of spontaneous breathing and protective reflexes was similar following the two drugs (McCleave & Blakemore, 1975).

(6)   Diazepam has been recommended for ECT (Gomez & Dally, 1975), but as it does not produce sleep in one arm–brain circulation time, it is not an anaesthetic induction agent. Diazepam is associated with more cardiac arrhythmias than methohexitone (Allen *et al*, 1980) and produces a slow and variable onset of sleep with a prolonged hangover effect.

(7)   Etomidate has been used for ECT as it has good cardiovascular stability and produces rapid recovery. It has similar characteristics to methohexitone (Gran *et al*, 1984), but its effects on adrenocortical function call into question its use for repeated anaesthesia.

(8)   Propofol produces smooth induction of anaesthesia followed by rapid and complete recovery. It can be painful on injection. Propofol attenuates the tachycardia and hypertension seen during ECT better than methohexitone, but it does not alter the incidence of cardiac arrhythmias (Rampton *et al*, 1989). Propofol reduces seizures by 40% and this probably contraindicates its use for ECT (Simpson *et al*, 1988; Rampton *et al*, 1989).

Muscle relaxants

(1)   Relaxant drugs are used to prevent forceful and potentially damaging convulsions, without totally ablating signs of muscle activity.

(2)   It is usual to remove dentures and insert a 'bite block' once the patient is asleep.

(3)   The patient's limbs should be protected during the seizure – all trolleys should be adequately padded.

(4)   Suxamethonium remains the agent of first choice in a dose of 0.5 mg/kg (Pitts *et al*, 1968; Konarzewski *et al*, 1988). Its action is terminated by the patient's plasma cholinesterase enzyme.

(5)   The dose of suxamethonium used and the seizure quality and duration must be recorded so that dosage can be optimised during the course of ECT. The seizure duration is inversely proportional to the dose of suxamethonium given (Miller *et al*, 1985).

(6)   The duration of action of suxamethonium is shortened by ECT (Bali, 1975) and is prolonged by lithium therapy (Martin & Kramer, 1982) although the latter effect is not clinically important.

(7)   Suxamethonium commonly causes myalgia, but the 2% incidence of muscle pains following ECT is less than the 70% expected, despite rapid ambulation (McCleave &

Blakemore, 1975). Suxamethonium is contraindicated in patients with certain muscle diseases, susceptibility to malignant hyperthermia, high plasma potassium concentration, upper airway obstruction and genetically determined or acquired lack of plasma cholinesterase.

(8)   If suxamethonium cannot be used for ECT then the depolarising relaxant mivacurium is probably the best option. This dose should be allowed adequate time to work.

Ventilation

(1)   The most important aspect of anaesthesia for ECT is the provision of oxygen.

(2)   Hypoxaemia does not augment treatment. It has been noted that "[cardiac] ectopic phenomena occurred almost uniformly during deepest cyanosis following a convulsion", and these could be corrected by administration of oxygen (Bankhead *et al*, 1950).

(3)   It has been suggested that oxygenation before ECT is unnecessary in healthy patients, as long as they are ventilated with room air following the convulsion (Woodruff *et al*, 1968). It has since been shown that hypoxaemia is a frequent problem during ECT if preoxygenation is not adequate (Swindells & Simpson, 1987). Therefore it is vital to administer oxygen to all patients before applying an ECT stimulus.

(4)   Anaesthesia, paralysis and ventilation increase seizure duration, but increasing oxygenation alone does not prolong convulsions (Bergsholm *et al*, 1984). Seizure duration is probably increased by ventilation and paralysis acting to reduce the carbon dioxide concentration in the brain.

(5)   Seizure duration was increased by 68% when the alveolar carbon dioxide concentration was reduced from 5 kPa to 2 kPa by hyperventilation of intubated patients (Bergsholm *et al*, 1984).

(6)   Seizure duration can also be increased by passive hyperventilation using a non-rebreathing system with a face mask (Chater & Simpson, 1988). Therefore adequate ventilation during ECT ensures oxygenation and can increase seizure duration.

Anaesthetic and monitoring equipment (see also Chapter 14)

(1)   The anaesthetic and recovery areas must be fully equipped and regularly checked. The responsibility for keeping equipment in good working order must be clearly defined. The anaesthetist should have adequately trained assistance during ECT sessions. It may become mandatory to employ operating department personnel, who have all undergone a specific training programme, but all staff who work in the ECT unit should have regular training, updating and practice in basic and advanced life support techniques. *The requirement for staff education cannot be overemphasised.*

(2)   All anaesthesia must be given on a tipping trolley, as it is vital to be able to place the patient in the head down position rapidly.

(3)   There is probably no need to have a complete anaesthetic machine in the ECT treatment unit, as the main requirements are a source of oxygen and suction.

(4)   Nitrous oxide and volatile anaesthetic agents are not usually necessary; however, if these are supplied adequate scavenging of waste gases must be installed to comply with safety regulations.

(5)   It may occasionally be necessary to keep a patient anaesthetised after ECT, for example, in the case of suxamethonium apnoea; this can be achieved using total intravenous techniques via a syringe pump.

(6)   There is no need to supply a mechanical ventilator to the treatment unit; any patient needing prolonged ventilation must be transferred to an intensive care unit.

(7)   As oxygenation during ECT is of paramount importance, the best monitor is probably a pulse oximeter; this is also the least disturbing for the patient as it only requires

the use of a small ear or finger clip.

(8)   A capnograph must be available as it is important to be able to detect end tidal carbon dioxide if faced with a difficult intubation.

(9)   Routine ECG monitoring is less practical, especially as patients are often dressed in everyday clothes, but an ECG machine must be immediately accessible, as must means of measuring the patient's blood pressure and temperature, and adequate resuscitation equipment, including a defibrillator.

(10) A standard box of drugs for use in the event of a cardiac arrest or medical emergency must be kept in the unit and regularly checked (see list, pages 40–41.)

(11) These should include: diazemuls, aminophylline, salbutamol, hydrocortisone, adrenaline, atropine, lignocaine, isoprenaline, verapamil, esmolol, nitrates, naloxone, dantrolene and 50% dextrose.

(12) A means of measuring blood glucose concentrations, a chest drain and central venous cannulae should be available in the ECT suite.

Recovery from anaesthesia

(1)   The recovery area must be of sufficient size, well staffed and equipped with adequate monitoring and resuscitation equipment. In 1981, one nurse was found to be responsible for five recovering patients in 21% of units in Britain (Pippard & Ellam, 1981). This level of staffing is not acceptable.

(2)   There should be one trained member of staff for each patient not in control of protective reflexes.

(3)   The anaesthetist and psychiatrist must remain within easy reach of the recovery area.

Patients must be nursed in the lateral position and their transcutaneous oxygen saturation, ventilation, heart rate and blood pressure must be monitored until stable. Patients usually resume spontaneous breathing and regain protective reflexes within a few minutes of the end of the seizure. Possible problems during the recovery period include airway obstruction, ventilatory depression, cardiac arrhythmias, hypertension, hypotension, emesis, aspiration of gastric contents, delayed return of consciousness, agitation, confusion and headache. In patients who are slow to recover, a cerebral event, prolonged seizure activity, lack of plasma cholinesterase or hypoglycaemia should be suspected. Once patients have fully recovered they should be given something to eat and drink and returned to the ward, preferably accompanied by a nurse with whom they are familiar.

References

ALLEN, R. E., PITTS, F. N. & SUMMERS, W. K. (1980) Drug modification of ECT – Methohexital and diazepam. *Biological Psychiatry*, **15**, 257–264.

AYD, F. J. (1961) Methohexital – a new anaesthetic for electroconvulsive therapy. *Diseases of the Nervous System*, **22**, 388–390.

BALI, I. M. (1975) The effect of modified electroconvulsive therapy on plasma potassium concentration. *British Journal of Anaesthesia*, **47**, 398–401.

BANKHEAD, A. J., TORRENS, J. K. & HARRIS, T. H. (1950) The anticipation and prevention of cardiac ectopic complications in electroconvulsive therapy – a clinical and electrocardiographic study. *American Journal of Psychiatry*, **106**, 911-917.

BERGSHOLM, P., GRAN, L. & BLEIE, H. (1984) Seizure duration in unilateral electroconvulsive therapy – the effect of hypocapnia induced by hyperventilation and the effect of ventilation with oxygen. *Acta Psychiatrica Scandanavica*, **69**, 121–128.

CHATER, S. N. & SIMPSON, K. H. (1988) Effect of hyperventilation on seizure duration in patients having electroconvulsive therapy. *British Journal of Anaesthesia*, **60**, 70–73.

EL GANZOURI, A. R., IVANOVITCH, A. D., BRAVERMAN, B., *et al* (1985) MAOIs – should they be discontinued pre-operatively? *Anesthesia and Analgesia*, **64**, 592–596.

GOMEZ, J. & DALLY, P. (1975) Intravenous tranquillisation with ECT. *British Journal of Psychiatry*, **127**, 609–611.

GRAN, L., BERGSHOLM, P. & BLEIE, H. (1984) Seizure duration in unilateral electroconvulsive therapy – a comparison of the anaesthetic agents etomidate, althesin and methohexitone. *Acta Psychiatrica Scandinavica,* **69**, 472–483.

GREENAN, J., DEWAR, M. & JONES, C. J. (1983) Intravenous glycopyrrolate and atropine in induction of anaesthesia – a comparison. *Journal of the Royal Society of Medicine,* **76**, 369–371.

JOHNSON, G. C. & SANTOS, A. B. (1983) More on ECT and malignant hyperpyrexia. *American Journal of Psychiatry,* **140**, 266.

KONARZEWSKI, W. H., MILOSAVLJEVIC, D., ROBINSON, M., *et al* (1988) Suxamethonium dosage in electroconvulsive therapy. *Anaesthesia,* **65**, 474–476.

MALCOLM, K. & PEET, M. (1989) ECT and old age. *British Journal of Psychiatry,* **155**, 713–714.

MALTBIE, A. A., WINGFIELD, R. S., VOLOW, M. R., *et al* (1980) Electroconvulsive therapy in the presence of a brain tumour. *Journal of Nervous and Mental Diseases,* **168**, 400–405.

MARTIN, B. A. & KRAMER, P. M. (1982) Clinical significance of the interaction between lithium and a neuromuscular blocker. *American Journal of Psychiatry,* **139**, 1326–1328.

MCCLEAVE, D. J. & BLAKEMORE, W. B . (1975) Anaesthesia for electroconvulsive therapy. *Anaesthesia and Intensive Care,* **3**, 250–256.

MILLER, A. L., FABER, R. A., HATCH, J. P., *et al* (1985) Factors affecting amnesia, seizure duration and efficacy of ECT. *American Journal of Psychiatry,* **142**, 692–696.

PIPPARD, J. (1992) Audit of ECT in two NHS regions. *British Journal of Psychiatry,* **160**, 621–638.

—— & ELLAM, L. (1981) Electroconvulsive treatment in Great Britain. *British Journal of Psychiatry,* **139**, 563–568.

PITTS, F. N., WOODRUFF, R. A., CRAIG, A. G., *et al* (1968) The drug modification of ECT. II: Succinyl choline dosage. *Archives of General Psychiatry,* **19**, 595–599.

RAMPTON, A. J., GRIFFIN, R. M., STUART, C. S., *et al* (1989) Comparison of methohexitone and propofol for ECT. *Anesthesiology,* **70**, 412–417.

RICH, C. L. & SMITH, N. T. (1981) Anaesthesia for electroconvulsive therapy – a psychiatric viewpoint. *Canadian Anaesthetists Society Journal,* **28**, 153–157.

SELVIN, B. L. (1987) Electroconvulsive therapy – 1987. *Anesthesiology,* **67**, 367–385.

SIMPSON, K. H., HALSALL, P. J., CARR, C. M. E., *et al* (1988) Propofol reduces seizure duration in patients having anaesthesia for ECT. *British Journal of Anaesthesia,* **1**, 343–344.

——, ——, SIDES, C., *et al* (1989) The use of lignocaine to reduce pain on injection of methohexitone during anaesthesia for ECT. *Anaesthesia,* **44**, 688–689.

STRÖMGREN, L. S., DAHL, J., FJELDBORG, N., *et al* (1980) Factors influencing seizure duration and number of seizures applied in unilateral electroconvulsive therapy – anaesthetics and benzodiazepines. *Acta Psychiatrica Scandinavica,* **62**, 158–165.

SWINDELLS, S. W. & SIMPSON, K. H. (1987) Oxygen saturation during electroconvulsive therapy. *British Journal of Psychiatry,* **150**, 685–687.

WOODRUFF, R. A., PITTS, F. N. & MCCLURE, J. N. (1968) The drug modification of ECT. I: Methohexital, thiopental and preoxygenation. *Archives of General Psychiatry,* **8**, 605–611.

WYANT, G. M. & MACDONALD, W. B. (1980) The role of atropine in electroconvulsive therapy. *Anaesthesia and Intensive Care,* **8**, 445–451.

16. ECT and drugs
S. Curran & C. P. Freeman

Benzodiazepines

Diazepine effects include seizure protection, but the underlying mechanism is poorly understood (King *et al*, 1987). Most of the work relating to seizure thresholds has been done in animals, and concentrates predominantly on diazepam. There has been very little work in human subjects and even less on the implications of this for ECT.

Strömgren *et al* (1980) showed that patients receiving concurrent benzodiazepine medication had shorter seizure durations than controls. Standish-Barry *et al* (1985) examined the effects of 10 mg of diazepam given the night before ECT in eight in-patients with major depression. Seizure duration was assessed in a blind fashion by a consultant clinical neurophysiologist. Each patient acted as his or her own control. Seizure duration, measured using an EEG, was significantly reduced by the administration of diazepam night sedation; the average reduction was 24 seconds. It has been subsequently reported that ECT may fail therapeutically if concomitant benzodiazepines are prescribed (Pettinati *et al*, 1990). Work on animals has confirmed similar results for lorazepam and clonazepam.

Medazolam (i.v. and in bolus dose) is useful for the rapid control of severe post-treatment agitation, an uncommon side-effect of ECT in some patients. Diazepam (i.v.) is appropriate for some patients who have very long seizures (i.e. more than two minutes of seizure activity or EEG recording of over 90 seconds of peripheral fitting).

Recommendations

(1) Benzodiazepines are powerful anticonvulsants. Wherever clinically possible, their prescription should be avoided during ECT.
(2) Even shorter-acting benzodiazepines are present in significant quantities the morning after their use for night sedation. Use non-benzodiazepine sedation if necessary.
(3) Patients who have regularly taken benzodiazepines may have a lowering of their fit threshold during the withdrawal phase. Long-established benzodiazepine use should not be stopped suddenly just a few days before ECT. If the dosage cannot be gradually reduced before ECT, it may be best to continue during ECT, perhaps in reduced dosage.
(4) Medazolam is useful in some patients who develop severe agitation in the recovery phase following an ECT treatment.

Tricyclic antidepressants (TCAs)

Seizures are among the most serious side-effects of psychotropic drugs (Markowitz & Brown, 1987). The incidence of seizures in patients on therapeutic doses of TCAs is approximately 4% (Betts *et al*, 1968). Tricyclic antidepressants have been associated with the occurrence of seizures both following overdose and after therapeutic administration. Seizures have been reported in patients both with and without a past history of seizures (Shannon *et al*, 1988; Wroblewski *et al*, 1990). Wroblewski *et al* (1990) examined retro-spectively the case histories of 68 brain-injured patients. The incidence of seizures after TCAs was estimated to be 19%. Foulke & Albertson (1987) examined a series of 102 patients and found that the seizure incidence was 9% in those taking an overdose of TCAs.

The incidence of seizures with amoxapine seems low. Jefferson (1984) reviewed three cases. One patient had been taking amoxapine 600 mg/day in addition to lithium (which also reduces the seizure threshold).

No studies have been published which specifically examine the relationship between seizure threshold/duration and TCAs in relation to ECT. Doxepin (Ojemann *et al*, 1983) and monoamine-oxidase inhibitors (Markowitz & Brown, 1987) may be the safest antidepressants for treating the depressed patient at risk of seizures. Viloxazine has also been reported to be associated with a low incidence of seizures (Edwards & Glen-Bott, 1984). Markowitz & Brown (1987) have reported that maprotiline and amoxapine are associated with a higher incidence of seizures at therapeutic doses.

Recommendations

(1)   Little is known about the combined effects of tricyclics and ECT on seizure threshold or cardiac function.
(2)   Although tricyclics can cause seizures in some patients, there is little evidence that they have a clinically significant effect on seizure threshold in ECT.
(3)   Given that most courses of ECT are completed within three to four weeks, it is probably best to continue with established antidepressants through the course, to provide adequate early prophylaxis after the course.
(4)   In elderly patients or patients with pre-existing cardiac disease, wherever possible use non-cardiotoxic antidepressants.
(5)   Doxepin may be the safest TCA for patients with a history of seizures who require ECT.

Selective serotonin reuptake inhibitors

Despite the enormous amount of interest being generated by the selective serotonin reuptake inhibitors (SSRIs), it is surprising that very few data are available in relation to ECT. In overdose these drugs may cause convulsions (Feighner & Boyer, 1991). In general, early clinical studies suggested that SSRIs were not associated with seizures (Cooper, 1988). More recent studies have indicated that seizures may occur especially following overdose. Most of these have been case reports of fluoxetine associated with seizures (Riddle *et al*, 1989; Ware & Stewart 1989; Weber, 1989).

There has also been a clinical study examining the relationship between fluoxetine and ECT (Gutierrez-Esteinou & Pope, 1989). The seizure durations were compared between 12 patients receiving ECT plus fluoxetine (20–140 mg/day) and 25 controls receiving ECT in the absence of fluoxetine. Both at the start of treatment and during treatment, the seizure duration was slightly longer in the fluoxetine group. In addition, the energy (in joules) required to elicit a seizure was slightly less in the fluoxetine group. However, the differences were not statistically significant. Interpretation was difficult because patients in the fluoxetine group were also receiving a variety of psychoactive drugs including benzodiazepines, trazodone, neuroleptics, pemoline and thyroxine. However, the results fit in with the general concept that drugs associated with seizures may be associated with slightly longer seizure durations.

Two other studies, Harsch & Haddox (1990) and Kellner & Bruno (1989) demonstrated that the ECT/fluoxetine combination is safe.

Fluvoxamine has been noted to be proconvulsive, but this may be less than many other antidepressants, especially TCAs. Krijzer *et al* (1984) examined the proconvulsive effects of several different antidepressants by comparing intravenous administration in rats. These were ranked starting with the most proconvulsive drugs: in decreasing order these were amitriptyline, mianserin, imipramine, desmethylimipramine, viloxazine, maprotiline, zimeldine, clovoxamine, and finally fluvoxamine.

Harmant *et al* (1990) examined fluvoxamine in a dose of 50–200 mg/day for at least four weeks in 35 patients with epilepsy. There was no change in the number of seizures or in their nature. The study, which also included EEG monitoring, suggested that fluvoxamine is not epileptogenic and does not appear to alter seizure threshold.

The available evidence suggests that paroxetine has little effect on seizure threshold. Rasmussen & Johnson (1990) reported an incidence of seizures of 0.1% in patients taking paroxetine compared with imipramine (0.3%), amitriptyline (0.3%), mianserin (0.6%) and clomipramine (1.0%). In addition, no convulsions have been reported following these drugs taken in overdose (Rasmussen & Johnson, 1990). Sedgwick *et al* (1987) examined the EEGs of 23 depressed patients taking paroxetine before and four weeks after treatment. No significant differences were observed between the paroxetine 30 mg/day and placebo groups. There have been no clinical trials to address specifically the interaction between ECT and paroxetine and caution is recommended by the drug manufacturer.

Information supplied by the manufacturer of sertraline suggests that it has only been associated with a very small number of seizures. However, no case reports have been published, and the relationship to seizure threshold/seizure duration and ECT is not known.

Despite these negative reports, the Special Committee on ECT has received a considerable number of concerned enquiries about lengthy seizure activity in patients on SSRIs or where SSRIs have recently been stopped. This has been supported by comments at our regular ECT courses. We have therefore decided to make the following recommendations:

(1) Numerous anecdotal reports suggest that there is a problem with these drugs and ECT.
(2) Young women with low fit thresholds may be most at risk.
(3) Prolonged fitting of 2–3 minutes has been reported.
(4) Reports have occurred with fluoxetine, paroxetine and sertraline.
(5) Because reports have occurred both on SSRIs and when they have recently been withdrawn, stopping drugs with shorter half-lives such as paroxetine and sertraline is only recommended if a washout period of two weeks can be acheived. Fluoxetine has a much longer half-life, and a 3–5 week washout would be required.
(6) In most clinical situations where ECT is being considered, such a long wait will not be good or safe clinical practice. We therefore recommend the following in patients premedicated with SSRIs:
    (a) The drugs should not be discontinued before starting ECT, unless a full washout, as above, can be achieved.
    (b) Start with a low treatment stimulus (50 mC)
    (c) Be aware of the potential for prolonged fitting.
    (d) Alert anaesthetist and nurses.
    (e) Have i.v. diazepam drawn up and a pre-arranged agreement for terminating the seizure (say, after 90 seconds).

Monoamine oxidase inhibitors

Monoamine oxidase inhibitors should be avoided during ECT because they increase the seizure threshold (Trimble, 1978) rather than because of the potential anaesthetic risk. It is difficult to know the clinical relevance of this with regard to ECT, but it is worth noting if short seizures are occurring. No information is yet available about ECT and moclobemide.

It is now generally accepted that such drugs do not necessarily need to be stopped before general anaesthetic, providing there are clear clinical indications that they should be continued. In most situations, if a course of ECT is being considered, this is probably because the patient has failed to respond to the antidepressant drug that he is currently taking. In such circumstances it is good clinical practice to discontinue the drug. If, however, there are good clinical reasons why a monoamine oxidase inhibitor should be continued while ECT is being given, then it is obviously very important that the anaesthetist is made fully aware of this. The anaesthetist should also be told of any drugs like monoamine oxidase inhibitors that were prescribed but have been stopped within two weeks of a course of ECT starting (Fink, 1979).

Recommendations

(1)   Monoamine oxidase inhibitors do not need to be discontinued before ECT.
(2)   The anaesthetist should be informed about such medication.
(3)   There is little information on their effect on seizure threshold or duration.
(4)   There is no information on ECT and moclobemide.

Lithium

Lithium appears to reduce the seizure threshold, and most of the animal work supports the idea, but there is little direct experimental evidence relating this to ECT practice. In toxic quantities lithium is known to be neurotoxic and to induce seizures (Association of the British Pharmaceutical Industry, 1991). The majority of reports have described transient convulsions, but there have been reports of persistent seizure activity in lithium intoxication (Mallakh & Lee, 1987). Lithium is also reported to be associated with more severe memory impairment when given concomantly with ECT (Ahmed & Stein, 1987). It has been suggested that the increase in memory impairment and atypical neurological findings in patients receiving ECT and lithium occur because lithium reduces the seizure threshold (Milstein & Small, 1988). Milstein & Small (1988) have suggested that patients should not have ECT and lithium together. However, if lithium decreases the seizure threshold, the increased incidence of cognitive impairment might be because the electrical stimulus during ECT exceeds the threshold by a greater amount (and may be avoided by reducing the electrical energy supplied to keep the seizure duration to approximately 30 seconds). Mallakh (1988) has reviewed the complications of lithium and ECT and has suggested that this area is contradictory and confusing. Mallakh (1988) notes that repeated ECT in patients taking lithium may cause a "toxic delirium". Conversely, Holden (1985) has reported that lithium has no observable effects on the EEG or the seizure threshold.

Recommendations

(1)   Concomitant lithium administration is not a contraindication to ECT, but precautions should be taken.
(2)   Start with a low stimulus (50 mC), especially in younger patients.
(3)   Titrate stimulus intensity to keep fits at around 30 seconds.
(4)   Monitor orientation and cognitive function particularly carefully as course progresses.

Beta-adrenoceptor antagonists (β-blockers)

There is very little data available on the effects of beta-adrenoceptor antagonists on seizure thresholds, and in particular their relationship to ECT. Weiner (1986) reviewed the area and concluded that propranolol in doses as low as 5 mg/kg results in an increase in seizure threshold which is proportional to the dose. They suggested that beta-blockers cause an increase in seizure threshold and reduce seizure duration, which may interfere with the therapeutic effects of ECT. Since β-blockers are commonly prescribed, this possible complication has potential clinical implications.

Recommendations

No special recommendations, as more information is required.

Neuroleptics

There is evidence that neuroleptics are generally proconvulsant (Hashem & Frey, 1988) and such action is an indirect measure of their effect on seizure threshold. This effect may be dose dependent. For example, droperidol (0.625 mg/kg) lowered the seizure threshold in mice; however, in high doses (2.5 mg/kg) the threshold was elevated. Promethazine had no effect on seizure thresholds at low dose, but elevated the seizure threshold at high doses (2 mg/kg).

No studies have examined the relationship between neuroleptics, ECT and seizure threshold. Available evidence suggests that fluphenazine and haloperidol are among the neuroleptics with the least potential to induce seizures. The seizure inducing potential of different neuroleptics has been reviewed (Markowitz & Brown, 1987). Most of the available data are based on haloperidol and chlorpromazine. Trifluperidol, haloperidol and chlorpromazine produce seizures in mice, but usually in doses much greater than used therapeutically (Lapin & Ryzov, 1990). In another animal study (Burke *et al*, 1990), thioridazine (10 mg/kg) and clozapine (10 mg/kg) produced convulsions in all the mice tested, possibly through a toxic action. Sulpiride and metoclopramide were also associated with an increased risk of seizures, but the doses were relatively higher, for example, sulpiride 50 mg/kg.

Clozapine has recently attracted considerable attention. It is a dibenzodiazepine derivative with a piperazinyl side chain. It has weak binding affinity for both dopamine (D1 and D2) receptors and potent binding affinity for 5-HT_{1A} and 5-HT_2 receptors. The wide-ranging affinity of most neuroleptics makes interpretation of experimental results difficult. Clozapine also has antihistaminic, anticholinergic and alpha-adrenergic antagonistic properties (Jann, 1991). It has been claimed to reduce the seizure threshold in a dose dependent manner (Jann, 1991).

Recommendations

(1) No special precautions are needed.
(2) In small doses, neurleptics are better for sedation than benzodiazepines.

L-tryptophan

L-tryptophan may shorten seizures, but little information is available because L-tryptophan is usually prescribed in combination with other drugs.

Anticonvulsants

It is important to understand the relationship between anticonvulsants and ECT, as this group of drugs is increasingly being prescribed for the treatment of depression (Small, 1990). It is clear from the literature that there are important differences between the main anticonvulsants in terms of their effect on seizure threshold and seizure duration. As with most of the psychotropic drugs, very little information is available in relation to the effect of anticonvulsants on seizure threshold during ECT. The majority of studies have been on animals.

Phenobarbitone increases the seizure threshold in animals (File & Wilks, 1990). When phenobarbitone is withdrawn, the seizure threshold is reduced below the baseline level and this reduction persists for between 24–72 hours.

Taub *et al* (1990) examined the effects of intravenous carbamazepine in cats with doses ranging from 0.2–20.0 mg/kg. Doses greater than 1.0 mg/kg had a pronounced and immediate effect of increasing the seizure threshold; in the range 5–20 mg/kg this was increased by a factor of approximately five. Carbamazepine reduced the duration of a seizure once it had occurred as demonstrated by electrocorticography. Similar findings were reported in a further study by Loscher & Honack (1991). Carbamazepine 20–40 mg/kg significantly increased the seizure threshold in rats. Loscher & Honack (1990) confirmed that carbamazepine increased the seizure threshold. However, it was found that seizure threshold was higher in animals given electroshocks with short intervals, compared with those given shocks at intervals of 1–3 days. Consequently, if the duration between electroshocks is small, the anticonvulsant effects of the electroshocks and carbamazepine are not additive but synergistic.

Sodium valproate (25 mg/kg) has been demonstrated to increase seizure threshold in animal models (Sharma *et al*, 1990). It is important to consider the effects not only of the prescribed drug but also of the various active metabolites. For example, E-delta-2-VAP is a pharmacologically active metabolite of sodium valproate. Not only does it increase the seizure threshold in rats but this increase is 2–3 times greater than that of sodium valproate (Semmes & Shen, 1991).

Little is known about the effects on, or interactions with, ECT for new anticonvulsants (e.g. vigabatrin, lamotrigine).

Recommendations

(1)   Anticonvulsants raise seizure threshold and shorten seizure duration.
(2)   High stimulus energies may be required.
(3)   If anticonvulsants are used for mood stabilisation, it is probably best to continue them during ECT.
(4)   If anticonvulsants are used in epilepsy, the effect of the drugs should be to return the seizure threshold to normal range.

Caffeine

The adenosine receptor A1 subtype in the rat cortex has been credited with an anticonvulsant action. Immediately after a single ECT treatment, brain adenosine levels are increased (Schultz & Lowenstein, 1978). An increase in adenosine A1 receptors leads to an increase in the seizure threshold. The administration of an adenosine antagonist such as caffeine before ECT, increases seizure duration. In a case study (Shapira *et al*, 1985) and in a controlled trial involving eight depressed patients (Shapira *et al*, 1987), caffeine sodium benzoate 500–2000 mg was administered intravenously ten minutes before ECT, and seizure duration was compared with that of a previous treatment unmodified by caffeine. Seizure duration was significantly increased in patients exposed to caffeine. The administration of caffeine was not associated with significant cardiovascular or other adverse effects. Hinkle *et al* (1987) confirmed these findings. However, there has been at least one report of adverse effects following intravenous caffeine in a 49-year-old man, which quickly returned to normal (Acevedo & Smith, 1988).

A larger randomised, double-blind, placebo-controlled pilot study of 40 depressed in-patients examined caffeine augmentation. It compared two techniques for maintaining eizure duration during pulse unilateral ECT; pre-treatment with intravenous caffeine, versus electrical stimulus intensity dosing. Both techniques effectively maintained seizure duration. However, with caffeine this was accomplished without an increase in the mean stimulus intensity over the course of the ECT. There were no differences between the two techniques in therapeutic outcome or cognitive side-effects from the ECT. Caffeine pretreatment was well tolerated (Coffey *et al*, 1990).

Lurie & Coffey (1990) examined the effects of pretreatment with intravenous caffeine in patients with severe medical illness. Nine depressed in-patients with major cardiovascular or other medical disease were examined. In all cases, caffeine pretreatment lengthened seizures and this was followed by clinical improvement. The caffeine-modified ECT treatment was well tolerated, and no clinically significant adverse events were reported. Caffeine appears to be most beneficial during the later stages of treatment when the seizure threshold has been increased by the cumulative effects of the ECT.

Recommendations

Caffeine augmentation is a useful strategy:

(1) when maximum settings on the ECT machine are producing an inadequate fit, as measured by clinical response.
(2) when maximum settings on the ECT machine are producing inadequate clinical responses despite fits of adequate duration and generalisation.
(3) when maximum or high settings on the ECT machine are producing unacceptable side-effects.

Nicotine

Few studies which specifically examine the relationship between nicotine and ECT have been published. In large quantities, nicotine is proconvulsive.

Alcohol

The anticonvulsant properties of alcohol and seizure activity following ethanol withdrawal are well described (Green *et al*, 1990). However, there have been no studies examining the relationship between seizure duration, seizure threshold and ethanol in patients receiving ECT.

Conclusions

(1) The majority of patients receiving ECT will be taking concomitant medication.
(2) Psychotropic and anaesthetic drugs have a significant effect on both seizure threshold and seizure duration during electroconvulsive therapy.
(3) Drugs which reduce the duration of seizure by increasing the seizure threshold may be associated with treatment failure.
(4) Alternatively, a larger number of ECT treatments may have to be administered to achieve the desired therapeutic effect. This situation should be avoided as it increases the risk to the patient receiving ECT.
(5) Despite the obvious importance of this area, few clinical studies have been undertaken. Most of the research has been done in animals, and particularly rats.
(6) Although this work has highlighted some important areas for further research, such studies should be treated with caution.
(7) The effects of psychotropic and anaesthetic drugs on the efficacy and safety of ECT are neglected areas of research. There is an urgent need to undertake clinical research; this has the best chance of being successful if a collaborative approach is adopted between psychiatrists and anaesthetists.

References

ACEVEDO, A. G. & SMITH, J. K. (1988) Adverse reaction to the use of caffeine in ECT. *American Journal of Psychiatry*, **145**, 529–530.

AHMED, S. K. & STEIN, G. S. (1987) Negative interaction between lithium and ECT. *British Journal of Psychiatry*, **151**, 419–420.

AKKAN, A. G., YILLAR, D. O., SKAZAN, E., *et al* (1989) The effect of propranolol on maximal electroshock seizures in mice. *International Journal of Clinical Pharmacology, Therapy and Toxicology*, **27**, 255–257.

ASSOCIATION OF THE BRITISH PHARMACEUTICAL INDUSTRY (1991) *Data sheet Compendium 1991–1992*. Datapharm Publications Limited.

BETTS, T. A., KALRA, P. L., COOPER, R., *et al* (1968) Epileptic fits as a probable side effect of amitriptyline. *Lancet*, **1**, 390–392.

BURKE, K., CHANDLER, C. J., STARR, B. S. *et al* (1990) Seizure promotion and protection by D-1 and D-2 dopaminergic drugs in the mouse. *Pharmacology, Biochemistry and Behaviour*, **36**, 729–733.

COFFEY, C. E., FIGIEL, G. S., WEINER, R. D., *et al* (1990) Caffeine augmentation of ECT. *American Journal of Psychiatry*, **147**, 579–585.

COOPER, G. L. (1988) The safety of fluoxetine – an update. *British Journal of Psychiatry*, **152**, 77–86.

EDWARDS, J. G. & GLEN-BOTT, M. (1984) Does viloxazine have epileptogenic properties? *Journal of Neurology, Neurosurgery and Psychiatry*, **47**, 960–964.

FEIGHNER, J. P. & BOYER, W. F.(1991) *Selective Serotonin Re-uptake Inhibitors: The Clinical Use of Citalopram, Fluoxetine, Fluvoxamine, Paroxetine and Sertraline*. Chichester: John Wiley.

FILE, S. E. & WILKS, L. J. (1990) Changes in seizure threshold and aggression during chronic treatment with three anticonvulsants and on drug withdrawal. *Psychopharmacology*, **100**, 237–242.

FINK, M. (1979) *Convulsive Therapy: Theory and Practice*. New York: Raven Press.

FOULKE, G. E. & ALBERTSON, T. E. (1987) QRS interval in tricyclic antidepressant overdosage: inaccuracy as a toxicity indicator in emergency settings. *Annals of Emergency Medicine*, **16**, 160–163.

GREEN, A. R., DAVIES, E. M., LITTLE, H. J., *et al* (1990) Actions of chlormethiazole in a model of ethanol withdrawal. *Psychopharmacology*, **102**, 239–242.

GUTIERREZ-ESTEINOU, R. & POPE, H. G. (1989) Does fluoxetine prolong electrically induced seizures? *Convulsive Therapy*, **5**, 344–348.

HARMANT, J., VAN RIJCKEVORSEL-HARMANT, K., DE BARSY, T. H., *et al* (1990) Fluvoxamine: an antidepressant with low (or no) epileptogenic effect. *Lancet*, **336**, 386.

HARSCH, H. H. & HADDOX, J. D. (1990) Electroconvulsive therapy and fluoxetine. *Convulsive Therapy*, **6**, 250–251.

HASHAM, A. & FREY, H. H. (1988) The effect of neuroleptics and heuroleptic/analgesic combinations on the sensitivity to seizures in mice. *Anaesthetist*, **37**, 631–635.

HINKLE, P. E., COFFEY, C. E., WEINER, R. D., *et al* (1987) Use of caffeine to lengthen seizures in ECT. *American Journal of Psychiatry*, **144**, 1143–1148.

HOLDEN, C. (1985) A guarded endorsement for shock therapy. *Science*, **228**, 1510.

JANN, M. W. (1991) Clozapine. *Pharmacotherapy*, **11**, 179–195.

JEFFERSON, J. W. (1984) Convulsions associated with amoxapine. *Journal of the American Medical Association*, **251**, 603–604.

KELLNER, C. H. & BRUNO, R. M. (1989) Fluoxetine and ECT. *Convulsive Therapy*, **5**, 367–368.

KING, P. H., SHIN, C., MANSBACH, H. H., *et al* (1987) Micro-injection of a benzodiazepine into the substantia nigra elevates kindled seizure threshold. *Brain Research*, **423**, 261–268.

KRIJZER, F., SNELDER, M. & BRADFORD, D. (1984) Comparison of the (pro)convulsive properties of fluvoxamine and clovoxamine with eight other antidepressants in an animal model. *Neuropsychobiology*, **12**, 249–254.

LAPIN, I. P. & RYZOV, I. V. (1990) Effect of catecholaminergic drugs on quinolinate- and kynurenine-induced seizures in mice. *Journal of Neural Transmission*, **82**, 55–65.

LOSCHER, W. & HONACK, D. (1991) Anticonvulsant and behavioural effects of two novel competitive N-methylo-D-aspartic acid receptor antagonists, CGP 39551, in the kindling model of epilepsy. Comparison with MK-801 and carbamazepine. *Journal of Pharmacology and Experimental Therapeutics*, **256**, 432–440.

LURIE, S. N. & COFFEY, C. E. (1990) Caffeine-modified electroconvulsive therapy in depressed in-patients with medical illness. *Journal of Clinical Psychiatry*, **51**, 154–157.

MALLAKH, R. S. (1988) Complications of concurrent lithium and electroconvulsive therapy: a review of clinical material and theoretical considerations. *Biological Psychiatry*, **23**, 595–601.

—— & LEE, R. H. (1987) Seizures and transient cognitive deterioration as sequelae of acute lithium intoxication. *Veterinary and Human Toxicology*, **29**, 143–145.

MARKOWITZ, J. C. & BROWN, R. P. (1987) Seizures with neuroleptics and antidepressants. *General Hospital Psychiatry*, **9**, 135–141.

MILSTEIN, V. & SMALL, J. G. (1988) Problems with lithium combined with ECT. *American Journal of Psychiatry*, **145**, 1178.

OJEMANN, L. M., FRIEL, P. N., TREJO, W. L., *et al* (1983) Effect of doxepin on seizure frequency in depressed epileptic patients. *Neurology*, **33**, 646–648.

PETTINATI, H. M., STEPHENS, S. M., WILLIS, K. M., *et al* (1990) Evidence for less improvement in depression in patients taking benzodiazepines during unilateral ECT. *American Journal of Psychiatry*, **147**, 1029–1035.

RASMUSSEN, J. G. C. & JOHNSON, A. M. (1990) Incidence of seizures during treatment with antidepressants, including the new selective serotonin re-uptake inhibitor, paroxetine. Presented at the 28th Scandinavian Congress of Neurology, Reykjavik.

RIDDLE, M. A., BROWN, M. & DZUBINSKI, D. (1989) Fluoxetine overdose in an adolescent. *Journal of the American Academy of Child and Adolescent Psychiatry*, **28**, 587–588.

SCHULTZ, V. & LOWENSTEIN, J. M. (1978) The purine nucleotide cycle. *Journal of Biological Chemistry*, **253**, 1938–1943.

SEDGWICK, E. M., CILASUN, J. & EDWARDS, G. (1987) Paroxetine and the electroencephalogram. *Journal of Psychopharmacology*, **1**, 31–34.

SEMMES, R. L. & SHEN, D. D. (1991) Comparative pharmacodynamics and brain distribution of E-delta-2-valproate and valproate in rats. *Epilepsia*, **32**, 232–241.

SHANNON, M., MEROLA, J. & LOVEJOY, F. H., Jr. (1988) Hypotension in severe tricyclic antidepressant overdose. *American Journal of Emergency Medicine*, **6**, 435–422.

SHAPIRA, B., ZOHAR, J., & NEWMAN, M. (1985) Potentiation of seizure length and clinical response to ECT by caffeine pretreatment. *Convulsive Therapy*, **1**, 58–60.

——, LERER, B., GILBOA, D., et al (1987) Facilitation of ECT by caffeine pretreatment. *American Journal of Psychiatry*, **144**, 9.

SHARMA, S. K., BEHARI, M., MAHESHWARI, M.C., et al (1990) Seizure susceptibility and intra-rectal sodium valproate induced recovery in developing undernourished rats. *Indian Journal of Medical Research*, **92**, 120–127.

SMALL, J. G. (1990) Anticonvulsants in affective disorders. *Psychopharmacology Bulletin*, **26**, 25–36.

STANDISH-BARRY, H.M., DEACON, V. & SNAITH, R.P. (1985) The relationship of concurrent benzodiazepine administration to seizure duration in ECT. *Acta Psychiatrica Scandinavica*, **71**, 269–271.

STROMGREN, L., DAHL, J., FJELDBEG, N., et al (1980) Factors influencing seizure duration and number of seizures applied in unilateral electroconvulsive therapy. *Acta Psychiatrica Scandinavica*, **62**, 158–165.

TAUB, E., LONDSTROM, S., KLEM, V., et al (1990) A new injectable carbamazepine solution: antiepileptic effects and pharmaceutical properties. *Epilepsy Research*, **7**, 59–64.

TRIMBLE, M. R. (1978) Non-monoamine oxidase inhibitor antidepressants and epilepsy: a review. *Epilepsia*, **19**, 241–250.

WARE, M. R. & STEWART, R. B. (1989) Seizures associated with fluoxetine therapy. *DICP Annals of Pharmacotherapy*, **23**, 428.

WEBER, J. J. (1989) Seizure activity associated with fluoxetine therapy. *Clinical Pharmacy*, **8**, 296–298.

WROBLEWSKI, B. A., McCOLGAN, K., SMITH, K., et al (1990) The incidence of seizures during tricyclic antidepressant drug treatment in the brain-injured population. *Journal of Clinical Psychopharmacology*, **10**, 124–128.

17. Prescribing

C. P. Freeman

A set number of treatments should not be prescribed. The patient should be assessed after each treatment to see if further ECT is necessary. A few patients respond dramatically to one or two ECT treatments and further applications are unnecessary. Some patients may need 12 or more treatments, although most respond to a course of between four and eight. There is evidence that older patients and men require more treatments. The response to the initial two treatments is highly correlated with the overall change at the end of the course.

Barton *et al* (1973) failed to show any significant prophylactic value in giving extra ECT after clinical recovery or improvement, in the hope of preventing relapse. They showed that if relapses do occur they tend to occur early, 69% developing within two weeks. It is important to monitor a patient's condition carefully for two or three weeks, but to give additional treatment only if symptoms recur. Continuation or maintenance ECT may be indicated in some cases (see Chapter 21).

The most difficult clinical decision is at what stage to abandon ECT if it is not relieving symptoms. Unfortunately, no clear guidance can be given as to how many treatments should be prescribed when no clinical response is seen. No research studies have addressed this issue. It is usual practice to stop after about eight properly administered treatments if there has been no change at all in the patient's symptoms. Some patients appear to show a brief response early in the course but relapse quickly. In such individuals it is worth giving up to 12 applications of ECT. These figures are meant only as guidelines. There can be no hard and fast rules about the number of treatments required or how long the course should be continued. This has to be a matter of individual clinical judgement.

One possible reason for failure to respond to ECT is that treatment applications may not have induced effective seizures. In 1992 (Pippard, 1992), approximately 1 in 4 treatment applications were considered to be of little or no therapeutic benefit, in that treatment applications failed to induce any seizure activity, or induced partial (focal or unilateral) or very short generalised (bilateral) seizures. Contributing factors included lack of competency on the part of the operator, ECT machines which did not generate a sufficiently intense stimulus even at maximum output settings, and 'fixed' dosing strategies (see Chapter 22 and Appendix VI). Before abandoning ECT on the basis of no clinical response, it is advisable to check the patient's ECT record to determine whether or not the apparent lack of clinical response could be attributed to inadequate ECT administration. See Chapter 19 for a description of what is considered to be an 'adequate' seizure (a seizure which is likely to be of therapeutic benefit).

Treatment should be given two or three times a week. Studies which have compared two times weekly with three times weekly show no advantage for more frequent treatment. Daily ECT should not be given. At present there is no evidence that daily ECT produces more rapid recovery, and the memory impairment is severe. Once-weekly ECT may be indicated for elderly patients with marked post-treatment confusion, or for patients who have brief manic episodes during the treatment. If a sustained manic change is induced then the course should be stopped.

The relapse rate following ECT is high, and it is important that adequate steps have been taken to provide continuing treatment such as prophylactic antidepressant drugs. The patient may have originally failed to respond to one or more antidepressants before being given ECT, but this does not mean that antidepressants will fail to provide an adequate continuing or preventative effect.

References

BARTON, J. L., MEHTA, S. & SNAITH, K. P. (1973) The prophylactic value of ECT in depressive illness. *Acta Psychiatrica Scandinavica*, **49**, 386–392.

PIPPARD, J. (1992) Audit of electroconvulsive treatment in two National Health Service regions. *British Journal of Psychiatry*, **160**, 621–637.

18. Electrode placement: unilateral versus bilateral

C. P. Freeman

There is still very active debate about whether unilateral ECT (UECT) or bilateral ECT (BECT) should be routinely recommended. There is no doubt that UECT is associated with subtantially less memory impairment than BECT, and that some patients treated with UECT may have no memory impairment. It is also clear that with brief-pulse low-energy stimuli, the memory impairment with BECT is less than with BECT using a sine-wave stimulation (Akkan *et al*, 1989).

Studies comparing BECT with UECT demonstrate that BECT is a more powerful antidepressant treatment, and that BECT is the method of choice for the treatment of severe depressive illness, especially where speed of action is important.

In recommending the routine use of BECT we are aware that it has been argued that it is possible to make UECT as effective as BECT when careful attention is paid to location of the stimulus electrode, contact of the electrodes/scalp interface, seizure monitoring and the stimulus dosage. However, a number of studies that have paid scrupulous attention to technique have still shown clear advantages for BECT. In our opinion, for routine clinical practice in busy ECT clinics a constant-current (brief-pulse) stimulus and BECT should be used.

Many of the earlier comparisons of UECT and BECT used high-energy sine-wave stimuli. More recent comparisons using lower energy brief-pulse stimuli have shown larger BECT/UECT differences. The study by d'Elia & Raotma (1975) reviewed many such sine-wave studies, and is widely quoted as evidence that UECT and BECT are equally effective. They compared 29 studies that had addressed this question. Unfortunately, they misidentified two studies. If corrections are made for these, their review shows that 15 of the studies reported the two methods to be equally effective, 13 reported an advantage for BECT and one an advantage for UECT. Studies published since that time have shown even greater advantages for BECT. These results are summarised by Abrams (1986). The evidence would seem to be that a greater proportion of depressed patients receiving BECT improve, that the percentage improvement is larger, and that fewer treatments are required for melancholic patients (Abrams *et al*, 1983). A more recent study (Abrams *et al*, 1991), again on melancholic patients, showed no difference between BECT and high-energy brief-pulse UECT with wide inter-electrode spacing. Other factors which should be considered are:

(1) age: older patients have a higher fit threshold and may respond better to BECT;
(2) sex: seizure threshold is 50–100% higher in men than in women and men may respond better to BECT;
(3) electrical stimulation: BECT may produce greater electrical stimulation to diencephalic (specifically hypothalamic) structures;
(4) prolactin release is increased more with BECT than with UECT, suggesting greater hypothalamic stimulation with BECT;
(5) cerebral metabolic activity: both cerebral blood flow and brain electrical mapping data show large differences between BECT and UECT;
(6) EEG post-ECT slow-wave activity is greater with BECT and markedly lateralised to the treatment side with UECT;
(7) the only double-blind controlled trial of ECT versus simulated ECT that failed to show a significant difference between the two treatments used UECT (Lambourn & Gill, 1978);
(8) although there is clear evidence that BECT produces more short-term memory impairment, no studies have compared the effects on remote memory of UECT versus BECT.

Summary

The choice between unilateral and bilateral electrode placement is still controversial. Having reviewed the topic, it is our opinion that the balance of evidence points to bilateral electrode placement being preferable in terms of speed of action and overall effectiveness, provided that brief-pulse stimulation is available. There is increasing evidence that this type of treatment is more effective, and with newer ECT machines using brief-pulse stimulation, the side-effects are less than they used to be. It is recommended that all ECT clinics should now use up-to-date constant-current machines. If, however, the older sine-wave machine is being used, then side-effects from the routine use of bilateral ECT will be much more marked. In these circumstances, it may well be appropriate to make unilateral ECT the normal treatment until a new machine can be obtained.

However, the choice is not a simple one. Many patients do respond to UECT and there are claims that the high-energy UECT is as effective as BECT while still having fewer side-effects. There is urgent need for further studies comparing BECT and high-energy UECT.

When to use unilateral ECT:

(1)   Where speed of response is less important.
(2)   Where there has been a previous good response to UECT.
(3)   Where minimising memory impairment is particularly important, e.g. out-patient ECT.

When to use bilateral ECT:

(1)   Where speed and completeness of response have priority.
(2)   Where unilateral ECT has failed.
(3)   Where previous BECT has produced a good response without undue short-term memory impairment.
(4)   Where determining cerebral dominance is difficult.

References

ABRAMS, R. (1986) Is unilateral electroconvulsive therapy really the treatment of choice in endogenous depression? In *Electroconvulsive Therapy: Clinical and Basic Research Issues* (eds S. Malitz & H. A. Sackeim). *Annals of the New York Academy of Sciences*, **462**, 50–55.

——, TAYLOR, M. A., FABER, R., *et al* (1983) Bilateral versus unilateral ECT: efficacy in melancholia. *American Journal of Psychiatry*, **140**, 463–465.

——, SWARTZ, C. M. & VEDAK, C. (1991) Antidepressant effects of high-dose unilateral electroconvulsive therapy. *Archives of General Psychiatry*, **48**, 746–748.

D'ELIA, G. & RAOTMA, H. (1975) Is unilateral ECT less effective than bilateral ECT? *British Journal of Psychiatry*, **126**, 83–89.

LAMBOURN, J. & GILL, D. (1978) A controlled comparison of simulated and real ECT. *British Journal of Psychiatry*, **133**, 514–519.

WEINER, R. D. (1986) Minimizing therapeutic differences between bilateral and unilateral nondominant ECT. *Convulsive Therapy*, **2**, 261–265.

19. Monitoring seizure activity

A. Scott & T. Lock

The aim of ECT is to induce generalised seizure activity in the brain by electrical stimulation. The typical seizure is characterised on the electroencephalogram (EEG) by widespread high frequency spike-waves ('polyspike activity') followed by slower (three per second) spike and wave complexes. Polyspike activity occurs during the latent and tonic phases of peripheral seizure activity, and 3 Hz spike-and-wave during the clonic stage (see Fig. 2). The minimum requirements of a therapeutic seizure have not been defined.

In the absence of the EEG recording, peripheral (i.e. motor) events provide indirect evidence of cerebral seizure activity. The purposes of seizure monitoring are to ensure that the desired cerebral seizure activity has been induced and to enable proper stimulus dosing.

The typical generalised convulsion has an initial tonic phase and then a longer clonic phase (i.e. rhythmic alternative contraction and relaxation of the muscles of the limbs on both sides of the body). There may be a delay in the onset of the tonic phase following the electrical stimulation, known as the latent phase. The treatment stimulus may fail to induce any visible peripheral motor activity, sometimes called a missed or failed seizure. Causes include: (a) no cerebral seizure activity, i.e. the stimulus has failed to induce a cerebral seizure; (b) an excessively high dose of muscle relaxant which completely attenuates motor activity; (c) machine failure or poor contact between the electrodes and the scalp, resulting in the patient not having received a stimulation or having received only a portion of the stimulation.

The treatment stimulus may induce a tonic contraction in the face and limbs, or a convulsion lasting only a few seconds involving only one part of the body, or one or more limbs on the same side of the body only – the so-called partial seizure. An ECT stimulus may cause contraction of facial muscles by a direct action on the temporalis muscles. Contraction of facial muscles during the passage of the stimulus should not be confused with the induced convulsion which often commences after an initial delay (i.e. the latent period). Partial seizures are of no therapeutic benefit.

In determining whether or not effective ECT has been administered, the treating psychiatrist must determine that widespread clonic muscular activity has occurred and the length of the convulsive activity must be timed. We recommend that timing begins at the end of the electrical stimulation and stops at the end of widespread, that is bilateral, convulsive activity. Some clinicians prefer to time to the last visible muscular contraction in any part of the body as well as to the end of bilateral muscular activity. The first edition of this book suggested that a clinically effective convulsion should last at least 25 seconds, and that restimulation should be carried out if the convulsion lasted less than 15 seconds. As was pointed out at the time, these were meant as approximate clinical guides, not firm recommendations, and more research was needed. It is now clear that the length of the convulsion is not reliably related to the therapeutic efficacy of treatment.

A useful working definition of an adequate seizure at the first treatment session for the vast majority of patients is:

(1) generalised (i.e. bilateral)
(2) commencing with a tonic phase, the onset of which may follow a latent period
(3) a clonic phase
(4) duration of 15 seconds or more peripherally, and/or 25 seconds or more on the EEG recording.

There exists a minority group of patients who respond well to ECT despite having short (i.e. less than 15 seconds) convulsions. The majority of patients will, however, have generalised convulsions lasting 15 seconds or more at the first treatment session if they are adequately stimulated. We recommend that the length of bilateral convulsive activity be timed for two important reasons:

(1) Brief generalised convulsions, particularly at the beginning of a course of ECT, are unlikely to be associated with the polyspike progressing to 3 Hz spike-and-wave EEG pattern which characterises a typical generalised seizure.
(2) Brief generalised convulsions, partial and missed seizures must prompt review of the stimulus dose and of the factors that influence the seizure threshold, as well as the dose of muscle relaxant used and whether or not adequate electrical contact was established.

Each ECT suite should have a policy about when to restimulate a patient after a brief convulsion, and by how much the stimulus should be increased. The policy should address the likely causes of brief, partial and missed seizures: (a) contact between the electrode and the scalp; (b) dose of muscle relaxant; (c) the stimulus 'dose' relative to the patient's seizure threshold. Restimulation will clearly be required when missed or partial seizures are observed. It is important, however, that high doses of muscle relaxant are excluded as a cause, and the cuff technique (see below) is recommended in this respect.

The rise in seizure threshold that occurs over a course of ECT can be detected by a progressive shortening of convulsions over successive treatments. The rate of this progression will be an important influence on decisions about stimulus dosing over a course of ECT. A marked reduction in the length of convulsions at successive treatments should prompt a review of factors that influence the seizure threshold, and may require an increase in stimulus dose at the subsequent treatment to ensure that the stimulation is clearly above the seizure threshold.

Cuff technique

This is a simple and underused technique to minimise the influence of muscle relaxant in the assessment of convulsive activity. Advantages include; (a) a means of excluding high doses of muscle relaxant as a cause of missed seizures; (b) patients may be completely paralysed if indicated (e.g. patients with bone and joint problems) – the anaesthetist can use a somewhat larger dose of relaxant and the convulsion can be observed in the isolated arm.

It involves isolating one forearm or leg by inflating a blood pressure cuff to above systolic pressure before the muscle relaxant is given. The isolated limb does not become paralysed and the seizure can easily be observed. It is important to pump the cuff well above systolic pressure to allow for the rise in blood pressure that occurs during seizure activity. If this is not done, muscle relaxant will leak into the limb, and because venous return is occluded, that limb will become selectively paralysed.

When unilateral ECT is given, the cuff should be applied to the ipsilateral forearm or ankle so that one can check that a bilateral convulsion has occurred.

As a simple safety procedure, a manometer stand that is separate from the treatment trolley should be used so that there is no possibility of the cuff remaining inflated when the patient is moved to the recovery room.

The cuff technique as originally described involves the cuff being deflated after all suxamethonium depolarisation muscle-twitching had stopped, and before the electrical stimulus was applied. It is now more usual for the cuff to remain inflated throughout treatment. The length of time the cuff is kept inflated should be kept to a minimum, particularly in the elderly, and the cuff should be deflated as soon as adequate convulsive activity has been confirmed.

Table 1. Methods of monitoring seizure activity

Method	Advantages	Disadvantages	Recommendation
Timing of convulsion	Simple. Cheap	May be confused with muscle contraction during stimulation. Heavily influenced by muscle relaxant. Underestimates cerebral seizure activity	Minimum requirement in all ECT suites
Cuff technique	Cheap. Unaffected by muscle relaxant	Cuff pressure needs continual maintenance. May be left inflated after ECT. Risk of trauma in frail patients. Risk of clotting in sickle-cell disease. Underestimates cerebral seizure activity	This simple technique ought to be used routinely. Useful to assess brief convulsions. Valuable when total paralysis is desirable
EEG	Most direct assessment of cerebral seizure activity. Can detect both focal and pro-longed seizures. Research. Heuristic: insight into seizure disorders in general	Cost (doubles the cost of an ECT machine, plus cost of consumables, e.g. disposable electrodes and graph paper). Requires most training and supervision. Single channel cannot detect focal seizures	Underused in the UK. Built-in two-channel EEG monitoring is presently only available on machines manufactured in the US

EEG monitoring

The most direct available means of measuring seizure activity in the brain itself is by electroencephalogram (EEG). EEG monitoring of ECT has undoubtedly been underused in the UK, and few clinicians have any experience of the technique. Reliable EEG monitoring has a major advantage in that it rarely underestimates the length of cerebral seizure activity. This is clinically important because the observation of a short convulsion may lead to immediate re-stimulation or increased electrical stimulation at the next treatment, which may increase the likelihood of adverse cognitive effects. EEG monitoring can also detect unusually prolonged cerebral seizure activity that is not associated with apparent convulsive muscular activity. Prolonged seizures lead to markedly increased adverse cognitive effects, and, if untreated, more serious consequences.

Reliable EEG monitoring is of value in the detection of prolonged cerebral seizure activity, has an important role in the clinical management of patients in whom convulsive activity is observed to be brief, and when it is desirable to completely paralyse the patient.

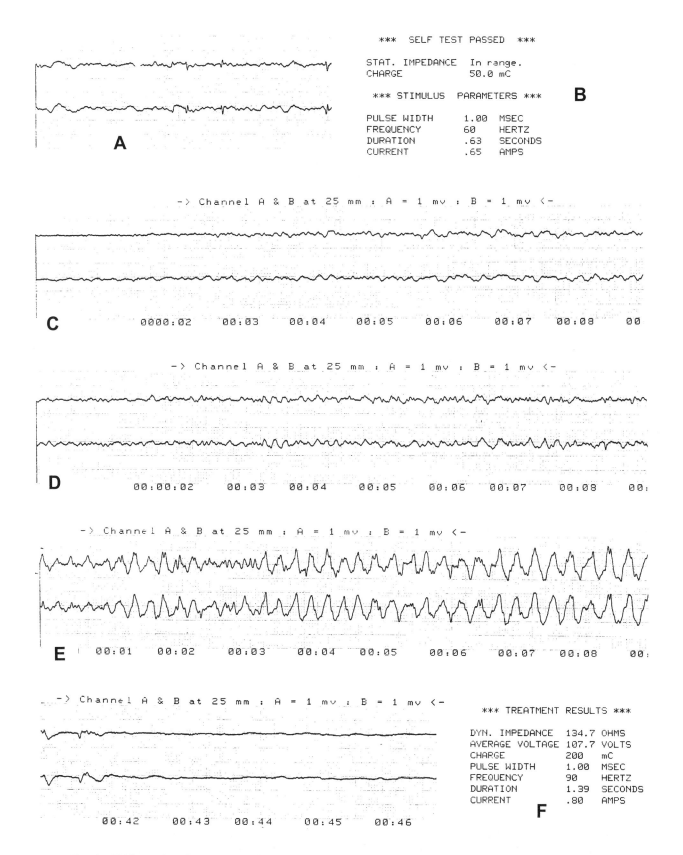

Fig. 1. EEG tracing from Mecta SR2 machine. A: baseline α rhythm, 8–12 Hz. B: self test result at setting for first stimulation (50 mC). C: First stimulation (50 mC), below seizure threshold. No peripheral muscle activity and no significant alteration in EEG pattern. D: Patient restimulated with 75 mC dose. Still no peripheral seizure activity and no significant alteration in EEG pattern. E: Patient restimulated with 200 mC dose, resulting in a generalised peripheral seizure lasting 22 seconds and EEG seizure activity lasting 41 seconds. F: Automatic printout at end of session, giving dose administered and stimulus parameters.

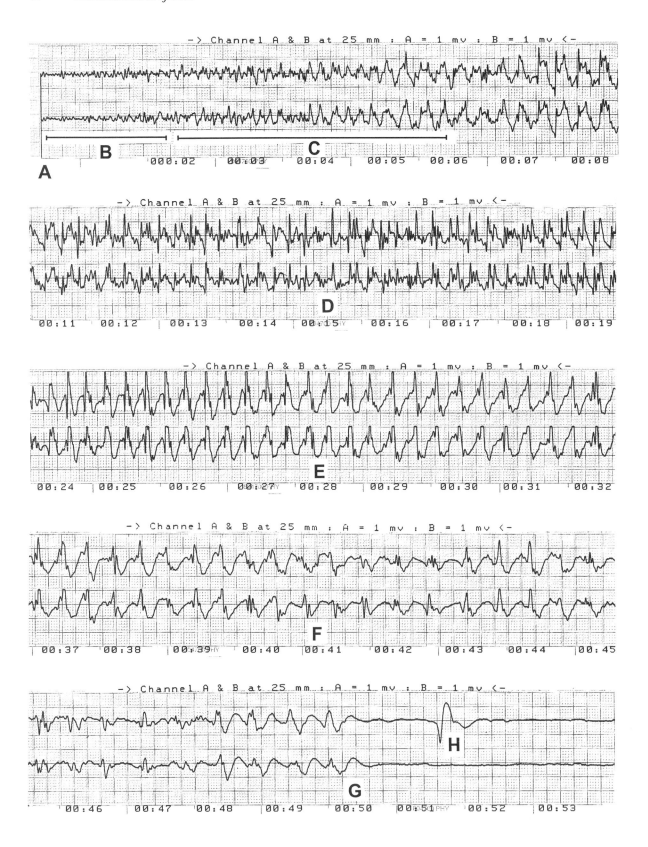

Fig. 2. EEG features of an 'adequate' generalised seizure. Compare left (top) and right (bottom) hemisphere tracings to confirm generalisation. A: end of electrical stimulation. B: latent phase – no peripheral seizure activity. Low amplitude, high frequency 'polyspike' EEG pattern. C: increasing amplitude of EEG polyspike, and gradual slowing of frequency. D: start of clonic phase of peripheral seizure. E: classic 3 Hz 'spike and wave' activity. F: gradual loss of spike and wave pattern. G: endpoint, after which EEG tracing has lower amplitude and frequency than at baseline (post-ictal EEG suppression). H: movement artefact; anaesthetist preparing to ventilate patient with oxygen.

20. Adverse effects of ECT

S. M. Benbow

Medical complications

Mortality

The mortality associated with ECT is thought to be similar to that of general anaesthesia in minor surgical procedures – approximately 2 deaths per 100 000 treatments . Despite the use of ECT for people with physical illnesses and at advanced ages, it is believed by many practitioners to carry a lower mortality than the use of antidepressant drugs (Weiner & Coffey, 1988). Cardiovascular complications are the main cause of mortality and morbidity, occurring immediately after the seizure or in the immediate recovery period. Since people with known cardiac disease are at greater risk of complications (Prudic *et al*, 1987), monitoring of this at-risk group during and for up to 15 minutes after treatment is advisable.

Prolonged seizures

If not terminated within three to five minutes, prolonged seizures may cause increased confusion and memory impairment. People on drug treatments which lower seizure threshold (for example, high-dose neuroleptics) will be at greater risk.

Spontaneous/tardive seizures

Spontaneous seizures following a course of ECT are rare, and occur no more commonly than in the untreated general population. Tardive seizures are defined as those seizures occurring following termination of the ECT induced seizure, and are also rare occurrences. When they occur in the immediate post-ictal period, motor evidence of seizure activity may be absent and the availability of EEG monitoring can be helpful in diagnosis.

Other medical side-effects

Immediately after treatment patients may experience headaches, muscular aches, nausea, drowsiness, weakness, anorexia and amenorrhoea (Gomez, 1975; Freeman & Kendell, 1986; Sackeim *et al*, 1987). Headache and nausea are not uncommon during and shortly after treatment, but are usually only mild and respond well to symptomatic treatments. If headache is severe, ibuprofen may be helpful (Abrams, 1992). Simple analgesics may be administered immediately after treatment if headache occurs recurrently (Burns & Stuart, 1991).

In the first week after ECT, memory problems and headache have been found to be the most prominent side-effects (Gomez, 1975; Freeman & Kendell, 1980; Baxter *et al*, 1986).

Rare adverse events

Aspiration pneumonia has been reported in modern ECT practice, in people with concurrent illnesses which increase their risk of gastroparesis, that is, loss of gastric muscle tone. Gastroparesis is likely in people with long-standing diabetes who have symptoms of peripheral and autonomic neuropathy, and should be suspected in people with hypothyroidism, amyloidosis, connective tissue disorders or gastric tumours (Zibrak *et al*, 1988). Aspiration of gastric contents using a nasogastric tube before anaesthesia may sometimes be necessary.

Ruptured bladder has also been reported in a man with prostatic obstruction (Irving & Drayson, 1984) and in another on a tricyclic who had failed to empty the bladder before treatment (O'Brien & Morgan, 1991).

Loose teeth, with the attendant possibility of fracture and inhalation, are a potential anaesthetic hazard (Faber, 1983).

Psychiatric complications

Some patients may switch into a manic illness during treatment with ECT. In these cases it may be unclear whether the diagnosis is of emergent mania or organic euphoric state. Detailed cognitive testing should help to differentiate the two. Some practitioners cease ECT and observe the person's affective state or start pharmacological treatments, but others continue ECT since it can be used as a treatment for mania as well as depressive illness.

Cognitive side-effects

Cognitive changes during and after a course of ECT have been extensively studied. The most common cognitive side-effects are memory impairment and confusion. It should be stressed, however, that many of the studies took place in the 1970s using machines which generated a sine-wave stimulus, which is known to be associated with more cognitive problems than brief-pulse stimulation, regardless of electrode placement (Weiner *et al*, 1986). Also, there was no attempt in the past to tailor the stimulus to the individual, and people with low seizure thresholds and those with high thresholds commonly received the same high stimuli. Modern machines allow stimuli to be individualised by using various regimes of stimulus dosing. Thus one would predict that with stimulus dosing and the new generation ECT machines, ECT should be associated with fewer cognitive side-effects than has been recorded in the British literature to date.

Memory impairment

Research studies, using several types of memory tests, have demonstrated that ECT may have an effect on several aspects of memory: memory for events which occurred before ECT (i.e. retrograde amnesia), both for the recent past or more distant past; and memory for events which take place after ECT (i.e. anterograde amnesia). Bilateral ECT has a greater effect on all aspects of memory compared with unilateral ECT, as does sine-wave stimulation compared with brief-pulse stimulation (Weiner *et al*, 1986). Memory impairment is cumulative, i.e. the effect on memory over a course of ECT increases. The evidence suggests that neither new learning nor memory for information from the past are permanently impaired. Objective memory impairment (on specific memory tests) is reversible. Some patients may, however, be left with discreet memory gaps for specific autobiographical events, the explanation for which is unclear.

Subjective memory complaints may differ from objective memory impairment (Freeman & Kendell, 1986). A common subjective complaint is memory loss for events immediately before, during or after a course of ECT. Many patients are unaware of memory difficulties, and some report an improvement of memory function after ECT. Severe depressive illness is itself associated with cognitive impairment, and some aspects of memory would be expected to improve if ECT effects the desired therapeutic response. A small number of patients treated with ECT in the past complain of persistent memory problems which are undetectable in objective memory tests: some patients within this group are likely to have chronic depressive symptoms.

Does ECT cause brain damage?

This was the subject of a very detailed review (Weiner, 1984) and a more recent study (Devenand *et al*, 1994). The conclusions of these two papers are best summarised in the author's own words:

> "ECT is not the devastating purveyor of wholesale brain damage that some of its detractors claim. For the typical individual receiving ECT, no detectable correlates of irreversible brain damage appear to occur. Still, there remains the possibility that either subtle, objectively undetectable persistent deficits, particularly in the area of autobiographic memory function, occur, or that a rarely occurring syndrome of more pervasive persistent deficits related to ECT use may be present."

We would endorse these conclusions.

Acute confusional states

Acute confusional states may occur between successive ECT treatments. People with pre-existing cognitive impairment, known neurological conditions or receiving concurrent psychotropic drug treatment are believed to be at greater risk. Patients who develop confusional states may be at greater risk of developing memory impairment. If a person develops an acute confusional state, the treatment technique should be reviewed to consider modifications which might lessen confusion, for example, increasing the interval between treatments, particularly in older people treated with bilateral ECT (Fraser & Glass, 1985), reducing the stimulus dose, or switching from bilateral to unilateral ECT.

Post-ictal delirium

Rarely, patients may develop post-ictal delirium with restlessness, agitation or aggression (Devanand *et al*, 1988) in the recovery phase. Although the episode resolves and is usually brief, it may recur with further treatments. Sympathetic nursing will be required, and sometimes restraint, or a fast-acting benzodiazepine (e.g. medazolam) will be needed (Litwack & Jones, 1988). At future treatments a low dose of a benzodiazepine can be given prophylactically as the patient recovers, immediately after ECT (Burns & Stuart, 1991).

Adverse psychological reactions

Adverse subjective reactions to ECT can be regarded as adverse side-effects of treatment. Prior to treatment people will often be anxious, but rarely a person develops intense fear of ECT during the course. The key to managing these reactions will be provision of support and information. During the consent process and throughout a course of treatment, patients and their relatives should be encouraged to express any anxieties and to seek information about treatment. Written information for the person concerned and their family may be helpful, but should not replace open discussion with staff. People who are also receiving, or have received, ECT can offer support and reassurance for one another. Some treatment clinics run group meetings for people receiving ECT and/or their close relatives.

Recommendations

(1)   People who are being asked to consent to ECT should be informed of any likely adverse effects of treatment.
(2)   Practitioners should monitor patients receiving ECT throughout the course, with particular attention to objective cognitive side-effects, medical complications and the patient's subjective experience of treatment side-effects.
(3)   If a person receiving ECT experiences any adverse effects, consideration should be given to modifying treatment technique or clinic procedure to minimise or ameliorate these effects.

References

ABRAMS, R. (1992) Technique of electroconvulsive therapy – theory. In *Electroconvulsive Therapy* (2nd edn), pp. 140–177. Oxford: Oxford University Press.

BAXTER, L. R. J., ROY-BYRNE, P., LISTON, E. H., *et al* (1986) Informing patients about electroconvulsive therapy – effects of a videotape presentation. *Convulsive Therapy,* **2**, 25–29.

BURNS, C. M. & STUART, G. W. (1991) Nursing care in electroconvulsive therapy. *Psychiatric Clinics of North America,* **14**, 971–984.

DEVANAND, D. P., SACKEIM, H. A., DECINA, P., *et al* (1988) The development of mania and organic euphoria during ECT. *Journal of Clinical Psychiatry,* **49**, 69–71.

——, DWORK, A. J., HUTCHINSON, E. R., *et al* (1994) Does ECT alter brain structure? *American Journal of Psychiatry,* **151**, 957–970.

FABER, R. (1983) Dental fracture during ECT. *American Journal of Psychiatry,* **140**, 1255–1256.

FRASER, R. M. & GLASS, I. B. (1985) Recovery from ECT in elderly patients. *British Journal of Psychiatry,* **146**, 520–524.

FREEMAN, C. P. L. & KENDELL, R. E. (1980) ECT. 1: Patients' experiences and attitudes. *British Journal of Psychiatry,* **137**, 8–16.

—— & —— (1986) Patients' experiences and attitudes to electroconvulsive therapy. *Annals of The New York Academy of Science,* **462**, 341–352.

GOMEZ, J. (1975) Subjective side effects of ECT. *British Journal of Psychiatry,* **127**, 609–611.

IRVING, A. D. & DRAYSON, A. M. (1984) Intraperitoneal rupture of the bladder and ECT. *British Medical Journal,* **288**, 194.

LITWACK, K. & JONES, E. E. (1988) Practical points in the care of the post-electroconvulsive therapy patient. *Journal of Post Anaesthesia Nursing,* **3**, 182–184.

O'BRIEN, P. D. & MORGAN, D. H. (1991) Bladder rupture during ECT. *Convulsive Therapy,* **7**, 56–59.

PRUDIC, J., SACKEIM, H. A., DECINA, P., *et al* (1987) Acute effects of ECT on cardiovascular functioning – relations to patient and treatment variables. *Acta Psychiatrica Scandinavica,* **75**, 344–351.

SACKEIM, H. A., ROSS, F., HOPKINS, N., *et al* (1987) Subjective side-effects acutely following ECT – associations with treatment modality and clinical response. *Convulsive Therapy,* **3**, 100–110.

WEINER, R. D. (1984) Does ECT cause brain damage? *The Brain and Behavioural Sciences,* **7**, 1–53.

——, ROGERS, H. J., DAVIDSON, J. R. T., *et al* (1986) Effects of stimulus parameters on cognitive side effects. *Annals of the New York Academy of Sciences,* **462**, 315–325.

—— & COFFEY, C. E. (1988) Indications for use of electroconvulsive therapy. *American Psychiatric Press Review of Psychiatry,* **7**, 458–481 (eds A. J. Frances & R. E. Hales). Washington, DC: APP.

ZIBRAK, J. D., JENSEN, W. A. & BLOOMINGDALE, K. (1988) Aspiration pneumonitis following ECT in patients with gastroparesis. *Biological Psychiatry,* **24**, 812–814.

21. Continuation ECT (maintenance ECT)

A. Scott

There has been a resurgence of interest in the use of ECT to prevent early relapse of an index episode of illness (continuation treatment) and to prevent future episodes of illness (maintenance treatment or prophylaxis). Unfortunately, there are few appropriate research findings to guide clinical practice. Most patients in descriptive studies of the use of continuation ECT suffer recurrent depressive illness.

An essential indication is that the acute episode of illness has shown a good response to ECT, either by way of a marked improvement or full recovery. Continuation ECT is often reserved for serious depressive illness, that is, associated with psychosis, suicide risk or marked self-neglect, where the illness has been resistant to treatment by antidepressant drug therapy, or where the patient was unable to tolerate such treatment because of adverse effects. Many contemporary reports concern older patients, but continuation ECT may be appropriate at any age.

The aim of continuation ECT is to maintain the patient's well-being with the minimum of physical risk and adverse cognitive effects. The frequency of treatment should be titrated to the needs of individual patients. Once the patient is markedly improved or symptom-free, continuation treatment may commence at weekly intervals, and the interval between treatments may be gradually extended up to fortnightly. Any re-emergence of depressive symptoms before the next treatment will require that the interval between treatments is reduced. The choice of electrode placement in continuation ECT is debated, but it is reasonable to use the placement associated with recovery during the index episode. Continuation ECT can be given without cumulative adverse cognitive effects using modern brief-pulse ECT machines. Nevertheless, memory must be assessed regularly throughout continuation treatment, the frequency of assessment being greater in older patients. The emergence of significant adverse cognitive effects would be an indication to use unilateral electrode placement. The impact of the use of concomitant psychotropic drug therapy on the efficacy of continuation ECT is unknown, but it would be good clinical practice to use the minimum, if any, concomitant drug therapy.

Continuation ECT can be given safely to out-patients, as long as the guidelines for day patient ECT are observed. There are no research data to determine what constitutes a sufficiently long course of continuation ECT. The only guidance we have is that 4–6 months would be considered the minimum if an antidepressant drug were being used as continuation treatment.

When ECT is used as a prophylactic treatment, it would be desirable to use a less frequent treatment schedule, for example, every 2–4 weeks, but the clinical response of the individual patient is the best guide in the absence of appropriate research.

Continuation ECT should be considered when:

(1) the index episode of illness responded well to ECT
(2) there is early relapse despite adequate continuation drug treatment, or an inability to tolerate continuation drug treatment
(3) the patient's attitude and circumstances are conducive to safe administration.

22. Stimulus dosing

T. Lock

The term stimulus dosing refers to the selection of the 'dose' of electricity used to induce seizures (see Chapter 23 for a description of the concept 'dose').

Pippard (1992) found that British ECT clinics used bilateral ECT almost exclusively, and that a 'standard' (fixed) dose was used to treat all patients at the first and subsequent treatment sessions. The standard dose was noted to vary up to four-fold from one clinic to another.

This section aims to review the scientific rationale for stimulus dosing, from which the reader will conclude that much contemporary British practice has not kept pace with research development.

Background

The scientific rationale for stimulus dosing originates in the findings of the Ottosson group (Ottosson, 1960) who undertook their research in the 1950s and 1960s when contemporary practice was to give bilateral ECT using a sine-wave ECT machine. They demonstrated that the therapeutic benefit of ECT derives from the induced fit, not the stimulus, and that the severity of cognitive side-effects was proportional to the dose of electricity used to induce the seizure. The latter finding provided the impetus for developments in ECT practice over the next two decades.

The 1960s and 1970s saw two important developments: the use of non-dominant unilateral ECT and brief-pulse ECT. Unilateral ECT, when used in conjunction with sine-wave stimulation, appeared to be as effective as bilateral ECT but was associated with fewer cognitive problems. Similarly, brief-pulse stimulation appeared to be as effective as sine-wave stimulation, but with fewer cognitive problems (Weaver *et al*, 1976, 1977; Weaver & Williams, 1982). In a memorandum published by the Royal College of Psychiatrists (1977), British psychiatrists were advised to use unilateral electrode placement and the minimum brief-pulse stimulus necessary for the induction of seizures.

British ECT clinics began to upgrade to constant current brief-pulse machines in the early 1980s: many re-equipped with Ectron Series 2 and Series 3 machines (see Appendix VI). What was not appreciated at the time was that, although grand mal seizures induced by brief-pulse unilateral ECT were clinically indistinguishable from those induced by bilateral brief-pulse or sine-wave ECT, therapeutic equivalency is dependent on the technique of administering unilateral ECT – in particular, on a wide separation of the electrodes, and on insuring that a relatively high suprathreshold dose is administered (Weiner *et al*, 1986). British psychiatrists adopted the Lancaster electrode position (Lancaster *et al*, 1958), where, unlike the d'Elia position (d'Elia 1970*a,b*; d'Elia & Raotma, 1975), the electrodes were not widely separated. Furthermore, it was not appreciated that the Ectron Series 2 and Series 3 machines were underpowered even at their maximum stimulus output setting.

In retrospect, it is not surprising that many British psychiatrists began to observe that unilateral ECT given with the then new brief-pulse machines (that is, Ectron Series 2 and Series 3) did not appear to be as effective as bilateral ECT using the old (Ectron Mark 4 sine-wave) machines (Lambourn & Gill, 1978). Many British psychiatrists spontaneously reverted back to using bilateral ECT (Pippard, 1988), and by 1989 the Royal College of Psychiatrists recommended that bilateral electrode placement be used almost exclusively (Royal College of Psychiatrists, 1989).

British clinical experience suggests that few patients now have profound or troublesome cognitive side-effects when bilateral ECT is administered by means of Ectron brief-pulse machines under existing stimulus dosing strategies. Why then alter existing ECT prescription and practice habits? Firstly, approximately one in four stimulations induce seizures which are unlikely to have a therapeutic effect (Pippard, 1992). Secondly, as British clinics re-equip with higher powered ECT machines, there is a risk of inducing unnecessarily severe cognitive side-effects if high-dose bilateral ECT is indiscriminately administered. Thirdly, because therapeutic equivalency can be achieved between unilateral and bilateral ECT, practitioners need to know about both methods and to select the most appropriate for each patient. Fourthly, even on existing schedules a few patients do complain bitterly of marked memory impairment and we must do all we can to minimise this.

Seizure threshold

The term seizure threshold refers to the minimum instrument setting required to induce a generalised seizure. Sackeim *et al* (1987*b*) using bilateral ECT and a brief pulse Mecta SR1 Machine, demonstrated that seizure threshold ranged between 25 and 800 millicoulombs or more in their patient population. This implies that there is a 40-fold inter-individual variation in seizure threshold. ECT is a powerful anticonvulsant, and seizure threshold rises by 25 to 200% during a course of treatment (Sackeim *et al*, 1987*b*, 1991).

Seizure threshold is affected by factors affecting electrical impedance (for example, electrode placement, the method of establishing contact between the electrodes and the scalp, the thickness of skin and bone), and the excitability of brain neurons (concurrent use of drugs with an anti-epileptic effect, including the general anaesthetic induction agent, anticonvulsant drugs, and blood oxygen and carbon dioxide saturation). The effects of a variety of factors on seizure threshold are summarised in Table 2. The new ECT record sheet contains a checklist of common factors which raise seizure threshold and/or shorten seizure duration, including age, sex, concurrent medications, and modality (that is, unilateral or bilateral electrode placement). In general, factors which raise seizure threshold tend also to shorten seizure duration, though some drugs (e.g. β-blockers) shorten seizure duration without altering seizure threshold. Factors which raise seizure threshold are additive in effect, for example, seizure threshold in an elderly man with little hair and a thick skull who is concurrently taking benzodiazepines and anticonvulsants is likely to be very high, while that of a young drug-free woman is likely to be low; seizure thresholds in drug-free elderly women, and young women concurrently taking benzo-diazepines and anticonvulsants, are likely to be somewhere between these two extremes.

It is important to appreciate that seizure activity can be induced in some brain regions more easily than in others – for example, sub-convulsive stimuli may induce seizure activity in deep limbic structures. Also, aberrant seizures (clonus of short duration) may be associated with EEG evidence of seizure activity in the frontal motor cortex, but not in other more posterior regions of cerebral cortex. If an ECT-induced seizure is to have a therapeutic effect, the stimulus administered must induce seizure activity throughout the whole brain; that is, the ECT stimulus must exceed the seizure threshold of the whole brain.

It is generally accepted that the most useful and valid measure of seizure threshold is in units of charge (millicoulombs, mC) (American Psychiatric Association, 1990), but seizure threshold may also be described in units of energy (Joules, J), stimulus intensity (mC/s), voltage (volts, V) or current (milliamperes, mA). Regardless of how seizure threshold is defined, it is important to recognise that it is not absolute. For example, with 'single-dial' machines (machines where output is defined in mC), seizure threshold may differ in the same individual if a different model of ECT machine is used. There is no agreement about an 'ideal' setting for brief-pulse stimulus parameters and different

Table 2. Factors affecting seizure threshold

Factor	Effect
Age	Raise
Anticonvulsants – concurrent or recently discontinued	Raise
Baldness	Raise
Barbiturates – concurrent or recently discontinued	Raise
Benzodiazepines – concurrent or recently discontinued	Raise
Bilateral electrode placement	Raise
Bones (thick), e.g. Pagets disease	Raise
Caffeine	Lower
Carbon dioxide saturation of blood (low)	Lower
Dehydration	Raise
ECT – increasing number of treatments	Raise
ECT – previous course within last month	Raise
Electrode contact with scalp (poor)	Raise
Hyperventilation	Lower
Methohexitone dose > 1.2 mg/kg	Raise
Methohexitone and ketamine in half doses	Lower
Oxygen saturation of blood (low)	Raise
Propofol	Raise
Sex (male)	Raise
Theophyllin	Lower

manufacturers have fixed different parameters. Furthermore, with 'multidial' machines (where the operator has control over four or more stimulus parameters), at a constant dose output (in mC), the dose may be below seizure threshold for one set of stimulus parameter settings, and above threshold with another set.

The therapeutic window

There appears to be a therapeutic window for the dose of stimulus (see Fig. 3). It is not the absolute dose which determines clinical response and the degree of cognitive side-effects, but the degree by which the dose exceeds seizure threshold. A dose marginally above seizure threshold will induce a generalised seizure, but the seizure may be of short duration and associated with evidence of incomplete generalisation and inadequate post-ictal suppression on an EEG recording. Particularly with unilateral ECT, marginally supra-threshold stimuli have a weak therapeutic effect (Sackeim *et al*, 1987*a*) and, regardless of electrode placement, marginally suprathreshold stimuli are associated with a slow clinical response (Robin & de Tiserra, 1982).

A dose below seizure threshold will fail to induce a generalised seizure; at best, the stimulation may induce cerebral seizure activity in a part of the brain which may manifest as unilateral clonus, or clonus of only a few muscle groups. Missed and partial (unilateral) seizures have no therapeutic effect. On the other hand, a dose greatly in excess of seizure threshold is likely to be associated with more severe cognitive side-effects without any therapeutic advantage. Regardless of electrode placement, the best results, in terms of maximising the therapeutic response and minimising the unwanted cognitive side-effects, are obtained with a 'moderately supra-threshold' dose, individualised to take into account the factors outlined above which affect seizure threshold. Furthermore, the amount by which the dose exceeds the threshold is critical in achieving therapeutic equivalency between unilateral and bilateral ECT, and the speed of response to ECT. Because of the

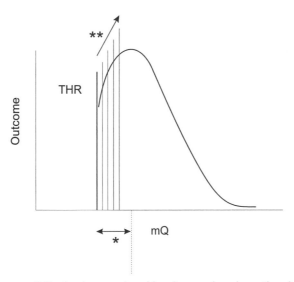

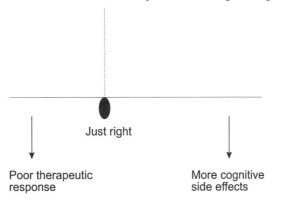

* Best outcome when 'dose' exceeds seizure threshold
  for a given individual by 50 to 100% for bilateral ECT (Sackeim, 1991)

** Seizure threshold rises by 80% on average during a course of ECT

Fig. 3. Seizure threshold and outcome – the therapeutic window (see text).

rise in seizure threshold after successive treatments, it is important to remember that the therapeutic window shifts to the right during a course of treatment, so the stimulus dose needs to be increased to maintain a consistent suprathreshold margin.

The problem is that therapeutic windows for unilateral and bilateral ECT (and for different models of ECT machine) have not been clearly defined. The general consensus is that a 'moderately suprathreshold' dose is between 50% and 200% above seizure threshold (that is, 1.5–3 times the threshold dose). An adequate dose for bilateral ECT is in the lower range (that is, 50–100% above threshold) while a higher suprathreshold dose (100–200%) is needed for unilateral ECT. Reports from Scandinavia where the Siemens 622 Konvulsator is used concluded that therapeutic results with unilateral ECT were as good as those with bilateral ECT. Abrams *et al* (1992), using a Thymatron machine, found no difference between unilateral and bilateral ECT in the symptomatic improvement of men using a fixed high-dose (378 mC) stimulus. There was, however, a non-significant trend towards faster improvement with bilateral ECT. At least one research group claim that therapeutic equivalency between unilateral and bilateral brief-pulse ECT may depend on a dose in excess of 200% above threshold (Sackeim, 1991; Sackeim *et al*, 1991).

Designing a stimulus dosing policy: general guidelines

(1) The primary consideration with stimulus dosing is to produce an adequate ictal response. Other considerations are minimising cognitive side-effects, and maximising the rate of clinical response.

(2) A dosing strategy should take into consideration the wide (40-fold) inter-individual variation in seizure threshold, factors affecting seizure threshold in a given individual, and the (25–200%) rise in seizure threshold in a given individual over successive treatments. Stimuli which are marginally suprathreshold are less therapeutic than stimuli in the recommended 'moderately suprathreshold' range, particularly for unilateral ECT. Grossly suprathreshold doses are associated with a greater degree of cognitive side-effects. It is the degree by which the dose exceeds threshold, not the absolute dose *per se*, which determines the degree of unwanted cognitive side-effects. Because of the rise in seizure threshold over successive treatments, most patients require one or more dose increases during the course of treatment in order to maintain a consistent suprathreshold margin.

(3) The decision to use unilateral or bilateral electrode placement should be based on an appraisal of advantages and disadvantages for each patient. If unilateral ECT is given, the electrodes should be widely separated (d'Elia, 1970*a*) and the stimulus dose in the high suprathreshold range. Because therapeutic equivalency of unilateral and bilateral ECT is dependant on a high standard of ECT administration, bilateral ECT is recommended where the expertise of those who administer ECT is in doubt.

(4) It is impossible to define a stimulus dosing policy for use in all ECT clinics and all patients; the key to success is flexibility. Each clinic should develop a local policy for the first and subsequent treatment sessions. Factors to consider are the model of ECT machine, the expertise of those who administer treatment, and the preferred electrode placement for the majority of patients.

(5) Regardless of the dosing strategy adopted at the first treatment session (see below), patients require restimulation if the initial stimulus dose has failed to induce an adequate seizure. Most modern machines have a 'self test' function which alerts the user to poor contact between the electrodes and the scalp, hence excessively high impedance. If this function is used routinely to establish the existence of adequate contact, an absent or aberrant seizure response to stimulation may be attributed to an insufficiently high stimulus dose. Therefore, if a patient needs to be restimulated, the dose should be increased by at least 50% for bilateral ECT and by at least 100% for unilateral ECT to ensure that the dose of the second stimulation is in the recommended moderately suprathreshold range.

(6) For patients who show a poor response to treatment and no more than mild cognitive side-effects, it is appropriate to:
    (a) increase the dose of the stimulus;
    (b) switch from unilateral to bilateral ECT (particularly if there is a poor response to four or more unilateral treatments).

(7) Seizure duration must not be used as the only indicator of seizure adequacy (see Chapter 19). Observed seizure duration is usually less than is shown by EEG recording, and therefore often less than the 25 seconds widely quoted as a guide to seizure adequacy. It is suggested that 15 seconds observed seizure may be taken as a guideline, but whether a seizure is "adequate" needs to be appraised in the context of many other factors which influence seizure duration, especially drugs and age. The crucial test is whether the patient is responding to treatment as expected. As a course of ECT proceeds there is a tendency for the seizures to become shorter. So long as the patient continues to improve at a satisfactory rate, this does not of itself require an increase in stimulus dose. Marked shortening of, or failure to elicit a seizure, and lack of progress towards recovery are useful indicators of the need to increase the stimulus to bring it again to moderately suprathreshold levels.

(8) Where patients have had adequate seizures but are experiencing marked cognitive side-effects, consider:
  (a) decreasing the dose of the stimulus
  (b) switching from bilateral to unilateral ECT
  (c) reducing the number of treatments administered per week (e.g. from two per week to one per week).

Dosing strategy at the first treatment session

There are two approaches:

(i) Selection of a predetermined dose. The predetermined dose must be known to be in the recommended moderately suprathreshold range for the majority (i.e. 80% or more) of patients (Abrams, 1992).

  e.g. Thymatron DG (Abrams, 1992)
      Unilateral electrode placement, adults 20–65 years old: 378 mC (75% of the maximum output of the machine).
      Unilateral ECT, adults over 65 years: 476 mC (95% of the maximum output of the machine).

The advantage of this approach is that it is simple. The main disadvantage is that the practitioner does not know by how much the dose exceeds seizure threshold in a given individual; if after subsequent treatments it is evident that the patient is not responding to treatment as expected, the practitioner still does not know whether the dose administered has been in the moderately suprathreshold range. Particularly with bilateral ECT, there is a risk of 'overdosing' patients with low seizure threshold and inducing excessive cognitive side-effects. The predetermined dose strategy is, therefore, best reserved for unilateral ECT with its lesser risk of cognitive side-effects.

Another disadvantage of this strategy is that limited information exists with respect to valid predetermined starting settings for different models of ECT machine; most importantly, practitioners are strongly advised to appraise critically the predetermined starting doses quoted by ECT machine manufacturers, as these may not be based on up to date research or audit data. Clinical audit and research are needed to establish appropriate starting settings for different models of ECT machines.

(ii) Dose titration. This entails administering a low stimulus which is likely to induce a seizure in only a small minority of patients; those patients who fail to have seizures are restimulated at successively higher doses, until a seizure is induced (Sackeim *et al*, 1987a). Once approximate seizure threshold is known, the dose is increased at the next treatment session to a level which is in the recommended 'moderately suprathreshold' range relative to the seizure threshold determined at the previous stimulus dosing session (that is, by about 50–100% for bilateral and 100–200% or more for unilateral ECT).

Regardless of electrode placement, the advantages of dose titration are that the practitioner knows with greater certainty that the dose administered is within the recommended suprathreshold range; that with bilateral ECT, the dose is not so high as to cause excessive cognitive side-effects; and that with unilateral ECT, the dose administered is sufficient for therapeutic equivalency with bilateral ECT.

The main disadvantage is that British psychiatrists and anaesthetists are unfamiliar with the technique, and some have expressed strong misgivings about the practical implications and the effects of inducing multiple sub-convulsive stimuli. Dose titration is widely employed in North American clinics, using a dose titration table which was originally developed for the Mecta SR1 machine; the table has since been adapted for use with the Thymatron DGx machine. Another disadvantage is that the majority of ECT machines at present in use in Britain (Ectron Series 5, Series 3 and Series 2 models) are unsuited to dose titration (see also Appendix VI). The original Neurotronic (Research version) machine likewise poses difficulties, as the operator needs to adjust four stimulus parameter output control dials in order to achieve small dose increments.

The four machines recommended by the Special Committee on ECT are all suitable for dose titration. Users of Mecta (British version) SR2 or JR2 machines and Thymatron DGx machines can draw on considerable North American clinical experience with equivalent American domestic models. Examples of dose titration are given below.

Example 1. Protocol for the Ectron 5A

Dr Allan Scott, ECT Department, Royal Edinburgh Hospital

General aims

(1)   To routinely measure the seizure threshold by an empirical titration method. An operational definition of the seizure threshold is "the minimum amount of electrical charge (in mC) that will induce a generalised tonic–clonic convulsion of at least 15 seconds at the first or second treatment in a course of ECT".

(2)   To adjust the dose of electrical charge to ensure that it is clearly suprathreshold, to maximise the efficacy of treatment, and yet avoid dosages that are grossly suprathreshold because this contributes unnecessarily to the adverse cognitive effects of treatment.

Titration of seizure threshold

(1)   *Patients not taking anticonvulsant drugs* (see Fig. 4)

The first stimulation at the first treatment will be routinely 50 mC. If an insufficient convulsion ensues, stimulation will be repeated with a dose of 75 mC. If an insufficient convulsion ensues after the second stimulation, the third stimulation should be increased

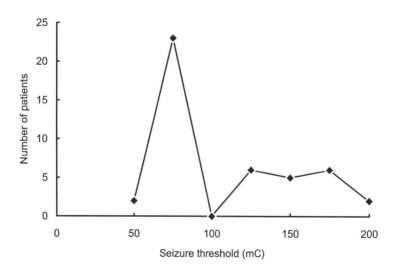

Fig. 4. Graph showing the seizure thresholds of 44 patients using the bilateral ECT technique described in Example 1. Note that for most patients, the seizure threshold is under 100 mC.

to 175 mC. (Very few patients free of anticonvulsant drugs will fail to have a convulsion with a dose of 175 mC at the first ECT.) Assuming that 175 mC led to a convulsion at the first treatment, the titration procedure can be continued at the second treatment by applying 100 mC at the first stimulation, and, if an insufficient convulsion ensures, increase the dose to 125 mC at the second stimulation. If still no adequate convulsion ensues, the third stimulation should be 225 mC for bilateral ECT and 375 mC for unilateral ECT. (The seizure threshold must be at least 150 mC.)

(2)   *Patients taking anticonvulsant drugs*
The absolute values and range of stimulation at the first treatment should be increased, that is, 100 mC, 200 mC and 300 mC. At the second treatment, the titration process can continue between the lower stimulation that did not lead to a convulsion and the higher stimulation that did.

Calculation of the seizure threshold

Ideally, the dose that did not induce a sufficient convulsion will be only 25 mC less than the dose that did. Although the actual seizure threshold will lie between these two values, it is sufficient to take the upper value as the seizure threshold (see worked example below).

Dosing strategy

(1)   For bilateral ECT, the dose should exceed the seizure threshold by 75 mC.
(2)   For unilateral ECT, the dose should be 2.5 times the seizure threshold.
(3)   The only exception to these general rules is the patient who had a sufficient convulsion with only 50 mC. It will be sufficient to increase the stimulation by 50 mC for bilateral ECT, and by 100% for unilateral ECT.

Seizure monitoring

(1)   It is the responsibility of the treating doctor to time the length of the generalised convulsion. The stop watch should be started at the end of electrical stimulation and stopped at the end of generalised, that is, bilateral clonic muscular activity.
(2)   During the titration process, stimulation should be repeated and increased (as above) until a generalised convulsion lasting at least 15 seconds is observed.
(3)   There is no simple relationship between the length of the convulsion and the therapeutic efficacy of treatment; nevertheless, timing of the convulsion is important because in an individual patient the progressive shortening of the convulsion is closely correlated with the rise in seizure threshold that occurs across a course of treatment.
(4)   Towards the end of a course of treatment in old patients and in patients treated with continuation or prophylactic ECT, it may never be possible to induce a convulsion lasting longer than 15 seconds because of the anticonvulsant effect of ECT.

Adjusting the dose throughout the course of treatment

Having established the seizure threshold and increased the dose accordingly at the second or third treatment, the likelihood is that the dose will have to be gradually increased by an average of 80% over a course of bilateral ECT as the seizure threshold rises. (This is to ensure that the dose remains clearly above the seizure threshold.) No hard and fast rules can be given except that there is no need to increase the dose unless there is a progressive shortening in the convulsion and that a marked shortening between two consecutive treatments ought to lead to an increased dose (25–50 mC) at the subsequent treatment.

A worked example of dose titration (bilateral ECT, no anticonvulsants)

Treatment	Stimulation	Convulsion	Comments
1	1. 50 mC	–	The seizure threshold (ST) lies between
	2. 75 mC	–	75 and 175 mC
	3. 175 mC	41 s generalised	
2	1. 100 mC	–	ST lies between 100 & 125 mC. Taken
	2. 125 mC	19 s generalised	as 125 mC
3	200 mC	45 s generalised	Dose = ST + 75 mC. The conv. induced
			by suprathreshold stimulation is longer
4	200 mC	43 s generalised	Note reduction in length of convulsion,
5	200 mC	38 s generalised	therefore detectable rise in seizure
6	200 mC	19 s generalised	threshold. Dose increased by 50 mC
7	250 mC	31 s generalised	

Termination of prolonged seizures

A prolonged seizure is one that lasts two minutes or more, and should be terminated immediately either by a further dose of induction agent or by intravenous diazepam. Prolonged seizures must be terminated promptly in consultation with the anaesthetist.

Example 2. Charge titration guidelines for the Neurotronic Therapy Systems

Dr K. W. de Pauw, St. James's University Hospital, Leeds

At the first treatment session start at Level 1 (180 mC) for *female* patients and at Level 2 (240 mC) for *male* patients. However, if a patient's previous ECT records indicate that a *higher* charge was required to achieve a satisfactory convulsion at the outset, adjust the frequency and time accordingly to the nearest charge level on the table.

In the event of an absent (a fit score of <2) or inadequate convulsion (a score of 2 but with a fit duration <25 seconds, calculated from the end of the stimulus to the cessation of *bilateral* convulsive activity), restimulate the patient after increasing the charge to the settings on the next level (e.g. from 180 to 240 mC). If the second application does not produce a satisfactory convulsion, restimulate the patient for the third time at the *next* level, anaesthetic conditions permitting. With a satisfactory convulsion, the charge at the second treatment session should be set at this level. Otherwise, increase the charge by one level, in the first instance. If unsuccessful, restimulate the patient for a second or third time at successive levels as already described.

Level	Charge (mC)	Current (mA)	Frequency (Hz)	Time (s)	Pulsewidth (ms)	Mode (uni/bi)
1	180	800	50	1.5	1.5	bi
2	240	800	50	2.0	1.5	bi
3	360	800	50	3.0	1.5	bi
4	720	800	100	3.0	1.5	bi
5	1080	800	100	4.5	1.5	bi
6	1440	800	100	6.0	1.5	bi

If, over successive treatment sessions during a course of ECT, the fit score remains 2 but seizure duration shortens markedly (e.g. from 25–30 to <20 seconds) increase the charge progressively at each session by one level (e.g. from 240 to 360 to 720 mC) to maintain an adequate fit length.

Key to fit score
0   No evidence of convulsion
1   Brief unilateral twitching
2   Definite bilateral convulsion
3   Inadequately modified bilateral convulsion

Charge (mC) = Current (A)* × Frequency (Hz) × Duration (s) × Pulsewidth (ms) × Mode**

   *   in amps, *not* milliamps, i.e. mA/1000 (e.g. 360 mA = 0.360 A).
   **   × 1 for uniphasic, or × 2 for biphasic current mode.

Note: these guidelines apply to all the Neurotronic Therapy systems, including the SLE NTS–R (but not the SLE NTS–C).

Example 3. The Neurotronic Therapy System machine (now SLE): bilateral ECT

Dr G. Fergusson, Argyll & Bute Hospital, Lochgilphead

Initial settings

Age range	Current		Other parameters
	Male	*Female*	
< 40 years	300 mA (135 mC)	200 mA (90 mC)	Frequency, 50 Hz; pulse
40–60 years	400 mA (180 mC)	300 mA (135 mC)	width, 1.5 ms; duration,
> 60 years	500 mA (225 mC)	400 mA (180 mC)	3 s; biphasic

Subsequent action (depending on the effects of the above)

Seizure	Action	Next ECT
> 60 seconds	Terminate if fit > 120 seconds	Reduce current by 100 mA
25–60 seconds	–	Maintain settings provided no significant cognitive side-effects
15–24 seconds	–	Increase current by 100 mA. Hold at this setting unless seizure falls below 10 seconds[1]
< 15 seconds	Restimulate once at +100 mA (after 20 seconds)	Continue at these increased settings for rest of course, unless seizure falls below 10 seconds[1]
Nil	Check machine/procedure. Restimulate. If still nil, increase by 100 mA and restimulate once more only	If still no fit, increase current by 100 mA and repeat procedure. Otherwise proceed as above

1. If seizure falls to less than 10 s during the ECT course as a result of the anticonvulsant action of the treatment, then increase the current by 50 mA at the next treatment to try to maintain an adequate seizure length.

(1)   The aim is to deliver a charge moderately above seizure threshold.

(2)   Increasing the current is the most effective way of inducing a seizure within a given total charge.

(3)   Should a current output of 800 mA be reached without the desired effect the next step is to increase the frequency to 100 Hz in order to increase the intensity of the charge. Following this the time can be increased in 0.5 s stages to a maximum of 6 s. It should never be necessary to increase the frequency to 150 Hz or to increase the pulse width above 1.5 ms.

(4)   If cognitive side-effects are troublesome and
    (a)   The seizure length was long – reduce current by 100 mA at next ECT.
    (b)   The seizure has been around 25 seconds – reduce the duration of the charge by 0.5 s at the next ECT treatment.
    (c)   The seizure has been short – increase the current by 100 mA and reduce the duration by 0.5 s at the next ECT treatment.

    OR   consider unilateral ECT

(5)   If there has been no clinical improvement after four apparently adequate treatments, then set the current at that which produced the first seizure activity and *increase* the frequency to 100 Hz.

(6)   The timing is taken from the end of stimulation to the end of bilateral seizure activity.

(7)   The above procedure may be reviewed in the light of continuing research.

Example 4. Stimulus dosing schedule for shortlisted models, based on the schedule for "USA domestic" Mecta SR1/JR1

Dr T. Lock, Broadoak Psychiatric Unit, North Mersey Community NHS Trust, Liverpool

Level		MECTA SR1/JR1					SR2/JR2	THY. DGx		ECTR. 5A
Suggested starting points		*Pulse width (ms)*	*Frequency (Hz)*	*Duration (s)*	*Current (A)*	*Charge (mC)*	*mC*	*%*	*mC*	*mC*
Female unilateral	1	1.0	40	0.50	0.8	32	25	5	25	25
Female bilateral/ male unilateral	2	1.0	40	0.75	0.8	48	50	10	50	50
Male bilateral	3	1.0	40	1.25	0.8	80	75	15	76	75
	4	1.0	40	2.00	0.8	128	125	25	126	125
	5	1.0	60	2.00	0.8	192	200	40	201	200
	6	1.0	90	2.00	0.8	288	275	55	277	275
	7	1.4	90	2.00	0.8	403	400	80	403	400
	8	2.0	90	2.00	0.8	576	550	100	504	550
	9						700	150	756	700
	10						1000	225	1008	

Values below double lines – machine in 'high range' (SR2/JR2) or 'Energy x 2' (DGx) modes.

MECTA (US Domestic version) SR1 and JR1 machines
Fixed biphasic brief-pulse waveform
Output range: 17–576 mC
Constant current: 550–800 mA; 6 steps
Frequency: 0.5–2 s; 6 steps

SR2/JR2 MECTA (British version) SR2 and JR2 models
Output in low range mode: 25 to 400 mQ
Output in high range mode: 450–1200 mQ
Control dial calibrated in 25 mQ steps (low range); 50 mQ steps (high range)

THY.DGx THYMATRON DGx model
Output in Standard mode: 25–504 mQ
Output in Flexidial mode: 50–1000 mQ
Control dial calibrated in % steps of maximum output in Standard and Flexidial modes

ECTR.5A ECTRON Series 5A model
Output range: 25–700 mQ
Control dial calibrated in 25 mQ steps

Stimulus dosing policy for first and subsequent treatment sessions

First treatment session

Aims
(1) To determine seizure threshold (ST): ST = the lowest dose (in mQ) which induces an 'adequate' seizure, defined by generalised peripheral tonic–clonic activity lasting 15 seconds and/or EEG polyspike, followed by 3Hz spike-and-wave activity lasting 25 seconds (i.e. generalised seizure 15/25 seconds).
(2) To determine the 'treatment dose' to be used at the next treatment session. Treatment dose = ST + 1 level for bilateral, or ST + 2 levels for unilateral electrode placement.
(3) To ensure that the patient has an adequate seizure.

Rules
(1) Always test for good contact between the electrodes and the scalp before stimulating the patient, and re-test if the electrodes are moved.
(2) Restimulate if a given stimulation results in:
    (a) a 'missed' seizure (no change in EEG pattern)
    (b) a partial seizure = focal peripheral activity and/or absence of generalised EEG polyspike/3Hz spike-and-wave activity.
    (c) generalised peripheral tonic–clonic activity lasting < 15 seconds and/or EEG polyspike/3Hz spike-and-wave activity lasting < 25 seconds.
    Note exception: a minority of patients have short but nevertheless adequate seizures.
(3) Always wait a minimum of 30 seconds between stimulations.
(4) Terminate seizures lasting two minutes or more by giving more general anaesthetic or intravenous diazepam. Warn the anaesthetist to prepare to do so after 90 seconds of seizure activity.

First stimulation
Start at the dose level for sex and electrode placement on the dose titration table for the appropriate machine. Start 1 level higher if
    (1) currently on benzodiazepines or anti-epileptics
    (2) ECT has been administered within the previous month
    (3) the patient is over the age of 65.

Accept as ST dose if seizure meets criteria for an 'adequate' seizure.

For treatment dose, go up 1 level from ST level at second treatment session for bilateral; 2 levels for unilateral.

If the patient is seriously ill, restimulate the patient with the 'treatment dose' at this session.

Second stimulation
If outcome of first stimulation does not meet criteria for adequate seizure, i.e. generalised peripheral seizure for < 15/25 seconds, partial or missed at first stimulation, wait 30 seconds, go up 1 level from ST level and *restimulate.*

Accept as ST dose if seizure meets criteria for an 'adequate' seizure.

For treatment dose, go up 1 level from seizure threshold level for bilateral at second treatment session; 2 levels for unilateral.

If the patient is seriously ill, restimulate the patient with the 'treatment dose' at this session.

NB. Exception: do not restimulate if the first two stimulations induce generalised peripheral tonic–clonic activity of less than 15/25 seconds, and the second seizure is shorter than or of equal duration to the first: assume first stimulation dose is the seizure threshold dose.

Third stimulation

If the outcome of the second stimulation does not meet the criteria for an 'adequate' seizure, wait 30 seconds, go up 2 levels and restimulate (i.e. skip 1 level).

If the stimulation now results in an adequate seizure, the ST dose could be the dose used or the previous (i.e. skipped) level. Therefore, at the second treatment session start with the skipped dose level to clarify the ST dose.

If three stimulations do not result in an adequate seizure, abandon the treatment session. At the next session, go up 1 level and continue titration – this is extremely uncommon.

Second treatment session

Where the ST dose has been determined, proceed with the treatment dose (approx. 90% of patients).
Where the ST dose has not been determined, continue with the titration procedure (approx. 10% of patients).

Third and subsequent treatment sessions

Seizure threshold rises as a course of ECT proceeds, and there is a tendency for seizures to become shorter. Increase the dose by 1 level if the duration of generalised seizures drops by 20% or more relative to the seizure duration at the second treatment session.

The clinical progress of the patient overrides seizure duration after the third treatment session: if the patient is experiencing severe cognitive side-effects, decrease the dose by 1 level, or switch to unilateral ECT. If the patient is not responding to treatment, increase the dose (by 1 level for bilateral; 2 levels for unilateral), or switch from unilateral to bilateral ECT.

Example 5. Duke University dosing schedule for Mecta SR1 and Thymatron

Initial and successive treatments (50% increments)

Level		MECTA SR1						THY. DGx (%)
		Pulse width (ms)	Frequency (Hz)	Duration (s)	Current (A)	Charge (mC)	Energy[1] (J)	
Female unilateral	1	1.0	40	0.50	0.8	32	5.6	5
Female bilateral/ male unilateral	2	1.0	40	0.75	0.8	48	8.4	10
Male bilateral	3	1.0	40	1.25	0.8	80	14.1	15
	4	1.0	40	2.00	0.8	128	22.5	20
	5	1.0	60	2.00	0.8	192	33.8	30
	6	1.0	90	2.00	0.8	288	50.7	50
	7	1.4	90	2.00	0.8	403	70.9	70
	8	2.0	90	2.00	0.8	576	101.4	100

1. Assuming 220 ohms dynamic impedance.

Instructions

Threshold determination
(1)   Start at level indicated by sex and electrode placement.
(2)   Increase level one step if restimulation is necessary.
(3)   If no adequate seizure after three stimulations at the first session, jump two levels for fourth stimulus, and, if successful, go one level lower for initial stimulus at second treatment session to continue titration.
(4)   If no adequate seizure after four stimulations at first session, abort treatment session and go one level higher for initial stimulus at second treatment session to continue titration.

Successive treatments
(1)   After establishing lowest level needed to produce an adequate seizure, increase two steps for next treatment with unilateral ECT and one step with bilateral ECT.
(2)   Use one step increments whenever any further increase in stimulus intensity is indicated because of missed, abortive, or inadequate seizure.

(3) Criteria for restimulation.
   (a) EEG seizure duration < 25 seconds
      Exceptions:
      (i) use 20 seconds cutoff after treatment 6 if patient > 60 years old.
      (ii) if there has already been two necessary increases within the past week, a 15 second criterion should be used.
   (b) Seizure morphology becomes less distinct (it is anticipated that this criterion will become more specific over time).

References

ABRAMS, R. (1992) *Electroconvulsive Therapy* (2nd edn). Oxford: Oxford University Press.

AMERICAN PSYCHIATRIC ASSOCIATION TASK FORCE ON ELECTROCONVULSIVE THERAPY (1990) *The Practice of Electroconvulsive Therapy – Recommendations for Treatment Training and Privileging*. Washington, DC: APA.

D'ELIA, G. (1970*a*) Unilateral electroconvulsive therapy. *Acta Psychiatrica Scandinavica*, **215** (suppl.), 5—98.

—— (1970*b*) Comparison of electroconvulsive therapy with unilateral and bilateral stimulation. II: Therapeutic efficacy in endogenous depression. *Acta Psychiatrica Scandinavica*, **215**, 30–43.

—— & RAOTMA, H. (1975) Is unilateral ECT less effective than bilateral ECT? *British Journal of Psychiatry*, **126**, 83–89.

LAMBOURN, J. & GILL, D. (1978) A controlled comparison of simulated and real ECT. *British Journal of Psychiatry*, **133**, 514–519.

LANCASTER, N. P., STEINERT, R. R. & FROST, I. (1958) Unilateral electro-convulsive therapy. *Journal of Mental Science*, **104**, 221–227.

OTTOSSON, J. O. (1960) Experimental studies of the mode of action of electroconvulsive therapy. *Acta Psychiatrica Scandinavica* (suppl. 145), 1–141.

PIPPARD, J. (1988) ECT custom and practice. *Psychiatric Bulletin*, **12**, 473–475.

—— (1992) Audit of electroconvulsive treatment in two National Health Service regions. *British Journal of Psychiatry*, **160**, 621–637.

ROBIN, A. & DE TISSERA, S. (1982) A double blind controlled comparison of the therapeutic effects of low and high energy electroconvulsive therapies. *British Journal of Psychiatry*, **141**, 357–366.

ROYAL COLLEGE OF PSYCHIATRISTS (1977) Memorandum on the use of electroconvulsive therapy. *British Journal of Psychiatry*, **131**, 261–272.

—— (1989) *The Practical Administration of ECT*. London: Gaskell.

SACKEIM, H. A. (1991) Optimizing unilateral electroconvulsive therapy. *Convulsive Therapy*, **7**, 201–212.

——, DECINA, P., KANZLER, M., *et al* (1987*a*) Effects of electrode placement on the efficacy of titrated low-dosage ECT. *American Journal of Psychiatry*, **144**, 1449–1455.

——, ——, PROHOVNIK, I., *et al* (1987*b*) Seizure threshold in electroconvulsive therapy – effects of sex, age, electrode placement and number of treatments. *Archives of General Psychiatry*, **44**, 355–360.

——, DEVANAND, D. P. & PRUDIC, J. (1991) Stimulus intensity seizure threshold and seizure duration. Impact on the efficacy and safety of electroconvulsive therapy. *Psychiatric Clinics of North America*, **14**, 803–843.

WEAVER, L. A., WILLIAMS, R. & RUSH, S. (1976) Current density in bilateral and unilateral ECT. *Biological Psychiatry*, **11**, 303–312.

——, IVES, J. O., WILLIAMS, R., *et al* (1977) A comparison of standard alternating current and low-energy brief-pulse electrotherapy. *Biological Psychiatry*, **12**, 525–543.

—— & WILLIAMS, R. (1982) The electroconvulsive therapy stimulus. In *Electroconvulsive Therapy – Biological Foundations and Clinical Applications* (eds R. Abrams & W. B. Essman), pp. 129–156. New York: SP Medical & Scientific.

WEINER, R. D., ROGERS, H. J., DAVIDSON, J. R. T., *et al* (1986) Effects of stimulus parameters on cognitive side effects. *Annals of the New York Academy of Science*, **462**, 315–325.

——, Devanand, D.P., Dwork, A.J., *et al* (1994) Does ECT alter brain structure? American Journal of Psychiatry, **151**, 957–970.

23. Electrical and neurophysiological principles
T. Lock

An understanding of electrical and neurophysiological principles relevant to the induction of seizures by electrical stimulation is important when operating ECT machines. This section should be read in conjunction with Chapter 22 and Appendix VI, since the manner in which an ECT machine is used is as important to the quality of ECT administration as the machine itself (Pippard, 1992).

Stimulus waveforms

During the first 40 years of its use, until the late 1970s, ECT machines delivered an alternating sine-wave stimulus at mains frequency and constant voltage. Newer machines deliver a constant current brief-pulse stimulus. Figure 5 shows one cycle of each of several stimulus waveforms, with current in milliamperes (mA) on the vertical axis and time, t, in milliseconds (ms) on the horizontal axis. A triangular waveform is a modified (chopped) sine waveform. Current flow may be unidirectional (that is, uniphasic) or bi-directional (biphasic). Figure 6 shows one cycle of the waveform generated by Ectron Series 5 and Series 5A machines.

Dose

In general terms, the area under the waveform curve represents the 'amount' (or 'dose') of electricity delivered per waveform cycle under a given load (that is, resistance, or impedance). The total amount of electricity delivered by a stimulation is the total area under the curve: this is equal to the area under the curve of one waveform cycle multiplied by the number of waveform cycles for the time that current flows (that is, for the duration of the stimulus: see Fig. 7).

The dose of electricity may be quantified in units of electrical charge, millicoulombs (mC) or electrical energy (joules, J). Charge is a measure of the total quantity of electrons delivered, while energy is a measure of the amount of heat dissipated as current flows.

Charge (mC) = Current × effective duration of current flow (milliamp-seconds (mAs))

Joules (J) = Voltage × current × duration of current flow (watt-seconds)

Ohm's Law states that: Voltage (V) = Current (A) × impedence (in ohms, or Ω)

Therefore:

$$\text{Joules (J)} = \text{Current} \times \text{current} \times \text{impedance} \times \text{duration of current flow}$$
$$(\text{Amps}^2 \times \text{impedance } (\Omega) \times \text{time (s)})$$

Energy (in J) may be converted to charge (in mC) as follows:

$$\text{Charge (mC)} = \frac{\text{Energy (J)}}{\text{Current (mA)} \times \text{impedance } (\Omega)}$$

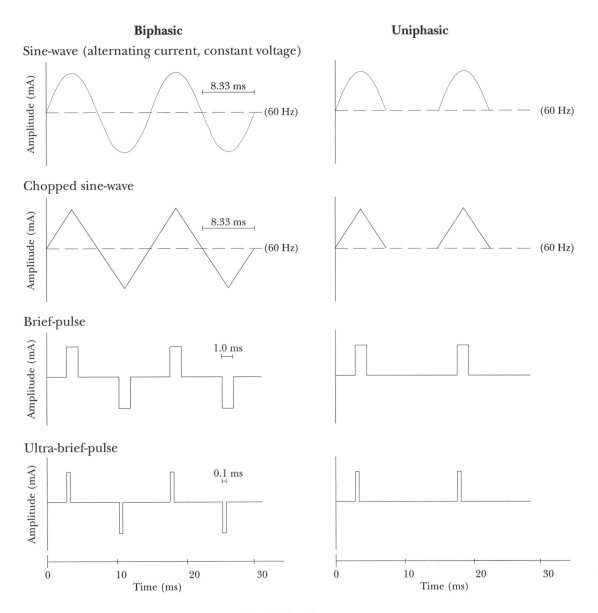

Fig. 5. Waveform types

Dynamic impedance values must be known for the calculation of electrical energy, but not for the calculation of charge. For constant current machines it is generally accepted that charge (mC) is the more useful and valid measure of 'dose'.

It is evident, with reference to Fig. 5 that if frequency, current and stimulus duration is the same for all waveform types, the 'dose' delivered by an ECT machine producing a sine waveform will be greater than that of a machine producing a triangular waveform, which in turn will be greater than that with a brief-pulse waveform, with the lowest dose being delivered by an ultra-brief-pulse machine. This is because of differences in the phase duration of the different waveforms.

Stimulus intensity

The term stimulus intensity is used to describe the peak current flow. A sine-wave stimulus is slow to reach peak stimulus intensity, whereas this is reached almost instantaneously

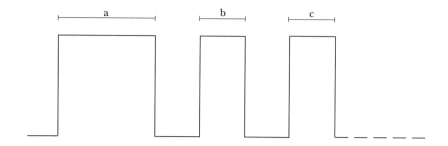

Fig. 6. One cycle of the uniphasic triple-pulse waveform generated by Ectron Series 5 and Series 5A machines. Pulse widths: a = 1.0 ms, b = 0.6 ms, c = 0.6 ms. Combined pulse width = 2.2 ms. Total phase width = 3.4 ms.

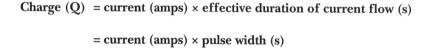

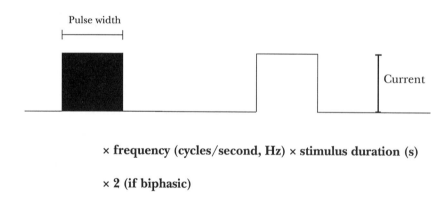

Fig. 7. Calculating electrical charge for brief-pulse current. Multiply current, in amps, (the height of the pulse) by pulse width (in milliseconds) to get the electrical charge of one pulse, in millicoulombs. (Current is usually quoted in milliamps, so remember to move the decimal point.) Now multiply frequency (the number of pulses per second) by the length of time that current flows (the duration of the stimulus in seconds) to give the total number of pulses administered to the patient. Multiply the total number of pulses by the charge of one pulse to give the total charge delivered to the patient, in millicoulombs. Multiply this figure by 2 if the ECT machine produces biphasic brief-pulse current.

with the brief-pulse waveform. The traditional sine-wave is a very inefficient way of depolarising neurons, and the stimulus intensity of a sine-wave stimulus needs to be in the order of two to three fold that of a brief-pulse stimulus. This is because a sine-wave is slow to reach peak intensity, and the stimulus intensity in the early (rising) part of the phase cycle is too low to depolarise neurons. After peak intensity has been reached, the sine-wave is slow to reach baseline (zero) intensity, and electrical charge or energy continues to be applied to neurons which may be in the depolarised, firing, or refractory phase. Much of the charge (or energy) of a sine-wave is therefore wasted. The configuration of the brief-pulse waveform is better suited to exciting neurons, and is therefore a more 'efficient' waveform (that is, seizures may be induced using significantly less electrical energy or charge).

Stimulus intensity is sometimes quoted in units of millicoulombs per second (mC/s). This concept of stimulus intensity is useful when comparing the output of one machine with another, or when comparing the output of one machine at different stimulus parameter settings (e.g. an output of 500 mC in 1 and 5 seconds gives, respectively, a stimulus intensity of 500 mC/s and 100 mC/s).

Constant current, constant voltage, or constant energy

ECT machines differ according to whether they operate on the principle of constant current, constant voltage or constant energy.

Constant current

Modern machines, (for example, Mecta, Thymatron, Neurotronic and Ectron Series 5A models) operate on the constant current principle. It will be seen from Ohms Law that an increase in impedance necessitates an increase in voltage if the predetermined current is to remain constant. Constant current machines automatically compensate for alterations in dynamic impedance in order to maintain the predetermined current intensity.

Constant voltage

Older models (for example, Ectron Mark 4 models) operate on the constant voltage principle. By Ohms Law, an increase in impedance will result in a decrease in current intensity if voltage remains constant. Under such conditions, the stimulus administered may fail to induce seizures. Conversely, if impedance is low the stimulus may be excessive. Constant voltage devices are now considered obsolete.

Constant energy

With constant energy devices, the user selects the energy to be delivered in joules. If voltage and current are fixed at a predetermined level, the only way the machine can compensate for an increase in impedance is by increasing the duration of stimulus. Under conditions of high impedance, the stimulus intensity may be too low to induce seizures regardless of the duration of the stimulation.

Dynamic and static impedance

The human head, in electrical terms, resembles a capacitor; brain tissue is a good conductor of electricity, so the dynamic impedance (that is, resistance to the flow of electricity) of brain tissue itself is negligible compared to that of the scalp (skin, bone and dura), which conducts electricity very poorly. When a treatment stimulus is passed, it must first overcome the static impedance of the scalp before current can flow through brain tissue. Impedance values drop dramatically during the first few milliseconds of the passage of an ECT stimulation.

Dynamic impedance can only be measured when current begins to flow; it cannot be measured in advance of applying the stimulus.

Constant current machines are designed to operate under an optimum 'load' (that is, dynamic impedance) and automatically alter voltage levels to compensate for alterations in impedance values, in order to maintain current at the predetermined level. For safety reasons, most machines are designed to limit the maximum voltage under conditions of high impedance. Obviously, if impedance is too high and the maximum voltage is limited, the current will not be maintained at the determined level, and the charge which is actually delivered to the patient may differ from the charge which the machine was set to deliver. A difference of 5% or less (that is, between predetermined and actual charge values) is acceptable.

The contact between stimulus electrodes and the scalp is the major determinant of static impedance; poor contact therefore results in high impedance values, high output voltages and a risk of skin burns and/or current levels which are too low to excite brain tissue. Loose connections (for example, between the electrode cables and the machine, or within hand-held electrodes) will also increase static impedance values. A difference of more than 5% between set and actually delivered charge values is indicative of excessively high static impedance, the most common cause of which is poor technique.

Modern machines should incorporate a test function which indicates whether static impedance is within the optimum range for that machine, and that it is safe to proceed with the actual electrical stimulation. The name given to this function differs from one manufacturer to the next. When this function is used, the ECT machine passes a small electric current between the electrodes which enables the machine to calculate the static impedance of the head.

The neurophysiology of seizure induction

A wide variety of pathophysiological states are able to produce seizures by virtue of the fact that they compromise neuronal membrane potential stability.

Spontaneous seizure disorders may be focal (or partial), where seizure activity remains localised to a particular region or lobe of the brain; secondary generalised partial seizures, where seizure activity has a focal onset but which then generalises (that is, spreads) to involve the whole brain; and primary idiopathic generalised epilepsy, where seizure activity involves the whole brain from the outset. ECT-induced seizures are of the secondary generalised type.

With ECT-induced seizures, the seizure focus is deliberately provided by an external source under controlled conditions, whereas with spontaneous seizures the seizure focus is 'internal'. The efficiency with which a given stimulus induces generalised cerebral seizure activity is determined by stimulus intensity relative to the area of tissue through which the stimulus is passing (that is, current density).

It is believed that the leading edge of each phase of the waveform is responsible for neuronal depolarisation (Weiner, 1980). It has also been suggested that the voltage of the stimulus must be sufficient to depolarise neurons, and that the charge (the quantity of electrons) must be sufficient to depolarise a sufficient number of neurons in order to overcome inhibitory influences (Swartz & Larson, 1989).

The ECT stimulus depolarises neurons in the path of the current flow between the two electrodes, generating bursts of high voltage 'spikes'. As the seizure discharge spreads to all parts of the brain by progressive depolarisation of surrounding neurons, it manifests peripherally as a motor convulsion, characterised initially by sustained contraction of all the muscles in the body with tonic rigidity and arrest of respiration – the 'tonic' phase of a generalised, major, or grand mal convulsion. After several seconds in that state, progressively longer bursts of neuronal inhibition develop in which the contracted muscles relax, resulting in alternating contraction and relaxation – the 'clonic' phase. Finally, inhibitory processes take over and the seizure is terminated. The muscle relaxant given prior to ECT attenuates much of the motor manifestation of induced seizures. A surface EEG recording of an ECT-induced generalised seizure is shown in Chapter 19. Missed seizures (that is, an absence of generalised seizure activity following stimulation) occur when the electrical stimulus fails to set into motion the neurophysiological events which result in generalisation of seizure activity throughout the brain. Partial or unilateral seizures occur when the stimulus is sufficient to excite neurons in a part of the brain, but insufficient to set into motion the train of events which result in generalisation of the cerebral seizure activity.

The therapeutic effect of ECT derives from the induction of a generalised seizure of adequate quality and duration, not from the electrical stimulus *per se.* Short generalised, missed, focal or unilateral seizures have little or no therapeutic effect. Generalised seizures, regardless of whether they are spontaneous or induced, are associated with a variety of alterations in brain function, for example, alterations in cerebral blood flow and metabolism, protein and other biosynthetic processes, membrane and neurotransmitter function. The fact that ECT may be effective when an adequate trial of antidepressants has failed suggests that several effects of seizures on brain function underlie the therapeutic efficacy of ECT.

It is unclear why, although generalised seizures induced by bilateral ECT are clinically indistinguishable from those induced by unilateral ECT, subtle differences exist in seizure quality. For example, unilaterally induced seizures are associated with less cerebral generalisation (Swartz & Larson, 1986), less post-ictal EEG suppression and/or lateralisation of post-ictal EEG suppression, a smaller endocrine response, and subtle differences in terms of therapeutic efficiency (Lambourn & Gill, 1978; Malitz *et al*, 1984). Although therapeutic equivalency may be achieved under certain circumstances (Weiner *et al*, 1986; Abrams *et al*, 1991), there is a statistically insignificant tendency towards a faster response with bilateral treatment, and a minority of patients will respond better (or will only respond) to the more intense stimulus offered by bilateral ECT.

Thus brief-pulse stimuli are more efficient at inducing seizures, whereas cognitive side-effects are more severe with sine-wave current and there is more profound post-ictal EEG disruption (Weiner *et al*, 1986), irrespective of electrode placement. Electrode placement and stimulus waveform exert independent and additive differential effects on cognitive function.

What remains unknown at present is the optimum configuration and duration of a brief-pulse stimulus with respect to maximising the efficiency of a given stimulus. Appendix VI summarises available information with respect to effective and/or safe minimum and maximum values for brief-pulse stimulus parameters.

References

ABRAMS, R., SWARTZ, C. & VEDAK, C. (1991) Antidepressant effects of high-dose right unilateral electroconvulsive therapy. *Archives of General Psychiatry*, **48**, 746–748.

LAMBOURN, J. & GILL, D. (1978) A controlled comparison of simulated and real ECT. *British Journal of Psychiatry*, **133**, 514–519.

MALITZ, S., SACKEIM, H. A., DECINA, P., *et al* (1984) Low dosage ECT – electrode placement and acute physiological and cognitive side effects. *American Journal of Social Psychiatry*, **4**, 47–53.

SWARTZ, C. M. & LARSON, G. (1986) Generalization of the effects of unilateral and bilateral ECT. *American Journal of Psychiatry*, **143**, 1040–1041.

—— & —— (1989) ECT stimulus duration and its efficacy. *Annals of Clinical Psychiatry*, **1**, 147–152.

WEINER, R. D. (1980) ECT and seizure threshold: effects of stimulus waveform and electrode placement. *Biological Psychiatry*, **15**, 225–241.

——, ROGERS, H. J., DAVIDSON, J. R. T., *et al* (1986) Effects of stimulus parameters on cognitive side effects. *Annals of New York Acadamy of Science*, **462**, 315–325.

24. Training and supervision

A. Scott

We recommend that a senior psychiatrist, preferably a consultant, should be responsible for the ECT clinic. The duties of the responsible psychiatrist can be divided into three main areas:

(1) to advise about appropriate treatment facilities;
(2) to develop a treatment policy;
(3) to train and supervise staff.

The clinic will require suitable treatment rooms, anaesthetic and resuscitation equipment, an ECT machine, appropriate nursing support and a rota of treating doctors. These matters will require liaison with hospital managers, nurses and anaesthetists.

The treatment policy should address pre-ECT assessment (in collaboration with anaesthetic colleagues), stimulus dosing, the method of routine seizure monitoring, and the protocols for the management of failed, partial or prolonged seizures. It will also be necessary to agree a standard treatment record form, consent form and information leaflet for patients (see Appendices).

The training and supervision of staff will be the most regular and time-consuming duties, and we recommend that the responsible clinician has dedicated time for these duties. We recommend that all psychiatric trainees have adequate training before they are asked to administer ECT. This should include the opportunity of seeing ECT administered by the responsible clinician, and personal supervision when treating patients. How each clinic is supervised will depend on local circumstances, but we recommend that wherever possible the administration of ECT should be restricted to psychiatric trainees as opposed to vocational trainees in general practice. Furthermore, it is desirable that the ECT rota is organised in such a way that continuity of patient care is maximised and that trainees have the opportunity of treating patients over several consecutive treatments. It is important that sufficient continuing supervision is available for junior doctors to ensure that clinical practice keeps pace with important research developments. Accordingly, the responsible clinician should have an active role in audit and academic teaching in ECT. Continuing education of the responsible clinician is important and should be supported by the employer.

Part III. The law and consent

25. ECT, the law and consent to treatment

J. Pippard & P. Taylor

In general, people with a psychiatric disorder can and should give valid consent to their treatment. Progression to treatment in the context of failure on the part of a doctor to give adequately balanced information to the patient about his/her disorder and the advantages and disadvantages of the proposed treatment could constitute legal liability on grounds of negligence. Treatment without consent could constitute battery.

It is widely recognised that some patients may be sufficiently impaired by their psychiatric disorder not to be capable of making valid decisions. British mental health laws recognise that capacity for decision-making may not be uniformly impaired so that, for example, capacity to decide about coming into hospital is, in law, treated as a separate matter from capacity to decide about some specific treatments or from capacity to manage money and affairs. ECT is one of the specific treatments for which the law prescribes a special process of consent in some circumstances.

Even among patients with severe mental disorder that may be most likely to benefit from ECT, the majority can make valid decisions about receiving it. Lidz *et al* (1984) reported on an empirical evaluation of informed consent in relation to ECT. Taylor (1983) reviewed some of the practical issues.

The common law, as it relates to consent to treatment, applies to all patients, informal or detained, except where statute specifically overrides it. Valid (real) consent is required before ECT may be given, unless common or statute law provides authority to treat without consent; in such a case the treatment must be:

(1) in the patient's best interest, i.e. necessary to save life or prevent a deterioration or ensure an improvement in physical or mental health;
(2) in accordance with a practice accepted at the time by a responsible body of medical opinion skilled in the treatment.

Consent must be freely given and based on an adequate understanding in broad terms of the purpose, nature, likely effects and risks of treatment, including the likelihood of its success and any alternatives to it, and of the likely consequences of not receiving it. The assessment of the patient's ability to decide about ECT and the nature and extent of the information to be given are matters for clinical judgement.

The patient should be told that consent may be withdrawn at any time and that fresh consent is then required before further treatment may be given.

Practice and regulations concerning consent to ECT are broadly similar throughout the United Kingdom. In England and Wales the relevant legislation is the Mental Health Act 1983; in Scotland the Mental Health (Scotland) Act 1984 and the Criminal Procedure (Scotland) Act 1975; in Northern Ireland the Mental Health (Northern Ireland) Order 1986. Consent to treatment in the Republic of Ireland is considered separately (see below).

(1) *The patient consents to ECT*

If the doctor is satisfied that real consent can be and has been given, the patient should be asked to sign a standard consent form, as suggested by the Department of Health and the defence societies. The doctor should also sign. The form is important evidence that consent has been sought, but not of the validity of that consent: this could be challenged, for example, on the grounds that the patient was not competent to consent or had not been given an adequate 'broad terms' explanation. It is, therefore, advisable to make a note in the case record of the interview at which consent was obtained. If the patient is detained under an appropriate section[1] the responsible medical officer, if satisfied that real consent has been given, is required[2] to certify, in the prescribed form, that the patient is capable of understanding the nature, purpose and likely effects of the treatment and has consented to it, before the treatment is started.

Consent should be for up to a limited and stated number of treatments, given during a stated time. Further consent should be sought and recorded if this number or time is exceeded or if, for any reason, there is a break in a series of treatments of more than three weeks, after which the treatment should be counted as a new course.

(2) *The patient refuses consent to ECT*

Alternative forms of treatment should be reconsidered.

ECT may not be given without consent to an informal patient who is capable of giving or withholding it. If there are strong indications for ECT, consider whether there are grounds for detaining the patient[3]. If the patient has been detained, the Commission[4] must be asked to arrange for an appointed doctor to visit to consider issuing a certificate, in the prescribed form[5], that "the patient is not capable of understanding the nature, purpose and likely effects of the treatment or has not consented to it but that, having regard to the likelihood of its alleviating or preventing a deterioration of his condition, the treatment should be given".

(3) *The patient is incapable of giving or withholding real consent*

A patient who resists treatment should be treated as if competent and refusing.

If a patient is not refusing ECT but cannot be said to be capable of giving real consent, there is an unresolved debate about whether it is legally necessary or in the patient's interest to detain such a patient in order to administer the treatment lawfully.

The legislation sets out a statutory regime with safeguards for patients and staff and lays down the circumstances in which ECT may be given to a non-consenting patient. Ordinarily, where a patient cannot consent to ECT the proper course of action is to use the relevant Mental Health Act.

It may sometimes be possible to proceed under the common law if the treatment is "in the patient's best interest" (c.f. paragraph 15.8 of the Mental Health Act Code of Practice (Department of Health & Welsh Office, 1990)). In these circumstances it is recommended that a second opinion be obtained from a consultant colleague who is not involved with the patient's treatment and that the situation be discussed with the patient's relatives. The decision is ultimately one for the professional judgment of the consultant who at all times must act reasonably.

(4) *ECT in an emergency*

    (a)   Informal patients: If the need for ECT is reasonably considered to be so urgent that any delay would be life-threatening, the treatment may be initiated under common law. Thereafter, proceed as in (3) above.

---

1. This does not include: (England and Wales) sections 4, 5(2), 5(4), 35, 37(4) 135, 136 or by direction under 37(4); (Scotland) sections 24, 25(1), 25(2), 117, 118; Criminal Procedure (Scotland) Act 1975 176 and 378; (Northern Ireland) articles 7(2), 7(3), 42, 129, 130 or by direction under 46(4).
2. (E and W) 58(3)(a); (S)98(3)(a); (NI) 64(3)(a).
3. (E and W) 2, 3; (S) 18, 26; (NI)4, 9.
4. (E and W) Mental Health Act Commission, (S) Mental Welfare Commission, (NI) Mental Health Commission for Northern Ireland.
5. (E and W) 58(3)(b) and 58(4); (S) 98(3)(b) and 98(4). (NI)64(3) (b) and 64(5).

(b) Detained patients: may[6] be given any treatment, including ECT, which is immediately necessary to save the patient's life or (not being irreversible) immediately necessary to prevent a serious deterioration of their condition; or (not being irreversible or hazardous) is immediately necessary to alleviate serious suffering by the patient; or (not being irreversible or hazardous) is immediately necessary and represents the minimum necessary to prevent the patient from behaving violently or being a danger to him/herself or to others.

If emergency ECT is given, the Commission should be informed so that a second opinion may be provided as soon as possible. Commission-appointed doctors usually attend promptly when asked so that it will rarely be necessary to use the legal provisions for urgent treatment or to give more than one ECT pending approval (or otherwise) for the rest of the course.

(5) *Involvement of relatives*

Except for a minor considered incapable of giving real consent, no relative may consent to the treatment of another person. It is good practice, if possible, to gain the cooperation of relatives or close friends in decisions about treatment. The patient should be fully informed that such approaches to relatives or friends are being made.

If the relatives disagree with the administration of ECT, but the consultant decides to give it, he/she is advised to make a record of the objections and of his/her reasons for proceeding with the treatment.

(6) *"Compulsory" ECT*

The opponents of ECT have recently been calling for a ban on compulsory ECT. Compulsory ECT is a confusing term and may lead to the false impression that psychiatrists are giving ECT to healthy individuals against their wishes. It is important to distinguish between this confusing use of the term and the use of ECT in detained patients. Many detained patients are able and willing to give their consent to ECT. If a detained patient is able to understand the nature, purpose and likely consequences of ECT and consents to it, then ECT can proceed. There is no justification for supporting a ban on ECT in detained patients. The severity of their illness which has led to their detention may well make them the patients who would need and benefit from ECT the most. Detained patients who refuse treatment or where there is any doubt about their ability and willingness to consent should be managed as in section (3) above.

Consent to treatment: Republic of Ireland

The Mental Treatment Act of 1945 (of the Republic of Ireland) does not deal specifically with treatment and consent, but it does pre-suppose the common law doctrine, and the elements of consent contained in the Law of Torts apply. In addition, precedents have been set by case law, which closely follows those established in English law.

For consent to be valid, there are three elements:

(1) the person must be competent to understand the implications of having or not having treatment;
(2) the person must give this consent freely, that is, free from coercion, fraud, etc;
(3) the person must be given adequate information. This is defined as what a reasonable doctor would tell his/her patient and implies that he/she would be informed of the

---

6. (E and W) 62; (S) 102; (NI) 68.

major common risks of the treatment. The adequacy of information is, therefore, determined by the standards of the profession as a whole.

If the patient is not competent to give consent and has been certified then treatment may be given. If the patient is incompetent but has not been certified then treatment may be given if there is genuine medical necessity for this. In practice, however, such patients are usually certified before treatment is given. There is a practice of getting the consent of relatives if the patient is incapable of giving consent, but there is no legal precedent for this.

Following a survey of ECT in the Republic of Ireland the following recommendations, which do not have legal status, were made in relation to the procedure where the validity of consent is in question:

(1) the consent form should be signed by an appropriate relative or guardian as well as by the patient;
(2) in cases where very ill patients refuse to accept treatment, a second consultant opinion is advisable following consultation with the patient's family.

References

DEPARTMENT OF HEALTH & WELSH OFFICE (1990) *Code of Practice.* London: HMSO.
LIDZ, C. W., MEISEL, A., ZERUBAVEL, E., *et al* (1984) *Informed Consent.* New York: Guilford Press.
TAYLOR, P. J. (1983) Consent, competency and ECT – a psychiatrists' view. *Journal of Medical Ethics,* **9**, 146–151.

Appendices*

I. A factsheet for you and your family

(Prepared by the Royal College of Psychiatrists' Special Committee on ECT)

Introduction

This leaflet will try to answer some of the questions you may have about ECT. You may wish to know, what is ECT? Why is it used? What is it like to have ECT and what are the risks and benefits?

When you are depressed it is often quite difficult to concentrate. Don't be concerned if you can't read through all of the leaflet. Just pick out the sections that seem important at the time, and come back to it later. You may wish to use it to help you to ask questions of staff, relatives or other patients.

Why is ECT used?

Most people who have ECT are suffering from depression. Although we have tablets for depression, some people do not recover completely and others take a long time. ECT is often used for these patients. In severe cases of depression ECT may be the best treatment and it can be life-saving.

Why has ECT been recommended for me?

ECT is given for many reasons. Some of the commoner ones are listed below. If you are not sure why you are being given ECT, don't be afraid to ask. It's sometimes difficult to remember things when you are depressed so you may need to ask several times.

* ECT is most commonly used to treat severe depression

* It may be helpful if you did not get better with antidepressant drugs

* It may help if you can't take antidepressant drugs because of the side-effects

* It may help if you have responded well to ECT in the past

* It may help if you feel so overwhelmed by your depression that it's difficult to function at all

What will actually happen when I have ECT?

For the treatment you should wear loose clothes, or nightclothes. You will be asked to remove any loose jewellery, hairslides or false teeth if you have them.

The treatment takes place in a separate room and only takes a few minutes. Other patients will not be able to see you having it. The anaesthetist will ask you to hold out your hand so you can be given an anaesthetic injection. It will make you go to sleep and cause your muscles to relax completely. You will be given some oxygen to breathe as you go off to sleep. Once you are fast asleep a small electric current is passed across your head and this causes a mild fit in the brain. There is little movement of your body because of

103

the relaxant injection that the anaesthetist gives. When you wake up you will be back in the waiting area. Once you are wide awake you will be offered a cup of tea.

What will happen immediately before the treatment?

An ECT treatment involves having an anaesthetic. You will need to fast (have nothing to eat and drink) from about midnight the night before each treatment. This will involve having no breakfast on the morning that you have ECT.

How will I feel immediately after ECT?

Some people wake up with no side-effects at all and simply feel very relaxed. Others may feel somewhat confused or have a headache. There will be a nurse with you when you wake up after the treatment to offer you reassurance and make you feel as comfortable as possible.

How does ECT work?

During ECT a small amount of electric current is sent to the brain. This current produces a seizure which affects the entire brain, including the centres which control thinking, mood, appetite and sleep. Repeated treatments alter chemical messages in the brain and bring them back to normal. This helps you begin to recover from your illness.

How well does ECT work?

Over eight out of ten depressed patients who receive ECT respond well, making ECT the most effective treatment for severe depression. People who have responded to ECT report it makes them feel "like themselves again" and "as if life was worth living again". Severely depressed patients will become more optimistic and less suicidal. Most patients recover their ability to work and lead a productive life after their depression has been treated with a course of ECT.

What is a course of ECT?

ECT is usually given two or three times a week. It is not possible to say exactly how many treatments you may need. Some people get better with as few as two or three treatment sessions, others may need as many as twelve and very occasionally more.

What ECT cannot do

The effects of ECT will relieve the symptoms of your depression but will not help all your problems. An episode of depression may produce problems with relationships, or problems at home or at work. These problems may still be present after your treatment and you may need further help with these. Hopefully, because the symptoms of your depression are better, you will be able to deal with these other problems more effectively.

What are the side-effects of ECT?

Some patients may be confused just after they awaken from the treatment and this generally clears up within an hour or so. Your memory of recent events may be upset and dates, names of friends, public events, addresses and telephone numbers may be temporarily forgotten. In most cases this memory loss goes away within a few days or weeks, although sometimes patients continue to experience memory problems for several months. ECT does not have any long-term effects on your memory or your intelligence.

Are there any serious risks from the treatment?

ECT is among the safest medical treatments given under general anaesthesia; the risk of death or serious injury with ECT is slight, about one in 50 000 treatments. For example, this is much lower than that reported for childbirth. Very rarely deaths do occur and these are usually because of heart problems. If you do have heart disease it may still be possible for you to have ECT safely with special precautions such as heart monitoring. Your doctor will ask another specialist to advise if there are grounds for concern.

What other treatments could I have?

Antidepressant drugs may be available to treat your particular condition and it is possible that some of them may work as well as ECT. The advantages will be discussed with you by your doctor.

Will I have to give my consent? Can I refuse to have ECT?

At some stage before the treatment you will be asked by your doctor to sign a consent form for ECT. If you sign the form you are agreeing to have up a certain number of treatments (usually six). Before you sign the form your doctor should explain what the treatment involves, and why you are having it, and should be available to answer any questions you may have about the treatment. You can refuse to have ECT and you may withdraw your consent at any time, even before the first treatment has been given. The consent form is not a legal document and does not commit you to have the treatment. It is a record that an explanation has been given to you and that you understand to your satisfaction what is going to happen to you. Withdrawal of your consent to ECT will not in any way alter your right to continued treatment with the best alternative methods available.

Are there any risks in not having ECT as recommended?

If you choose not to accept your doctor's recommendation to have ECT, you may experience a longer and more severe period of illness and disability than might otherwise have been the case. The alternative is drug therapy which also has risks and complications, and drug treatment is not necessarily safer than ECT.

II. Additional information for out-patients receiving ECT

This factsheet provides extra information, for patients receiving ECT as an out-patient. It should be read along with the general factsheet.

If you are having the treatment as an out-patient, there are some rules which must be followed because you will have a brief anaesthetic which will be given by injection into a vein in your arm.

* You must not have anything to eat or drink after midnight on the day before your treatment.

* If you are taking tablets in the morning, don't take them on the morning of your treatment; bring them with you and give them to the nurse who will give them to you with your cup of tea after the treatment.

* If you develop a severe head cold during the course of your treatment you may not be able to have an anaesthetic on a day when the cold is very bad: so ask someone to telephone and you will be told on which day you should next come. The telephone number is . . . .

* You must not drive a car or any motor vehicle on the day on which you have a treatment.

* Ambulance transport can be arranged, but it would be best if a relative or friend can drive you to the hospital and take you home again. You should arrive before . . . and will be ready to go home again around . . . (times will depend on clinic policy).

* You should not travel unaccompanied.

* You should not return to an empty house. Therefore if transport is arranged for you, please arrange for a relative or neighbour to be at your home when you return.

ECT is not an unpleasant treatment, although you may have a slight 'muzzy' feeling or headache after you wake up from the anaesthetic; this generally passes off after you have drunk a cup of tea which the nurse will bring you.

The treatment does not have an immediate effect so don't be worried if you do not feel better after the first few treatments. If you wish to discuss your progress with your doctor before any of your treatment sessions, let the nurse know when you arrive.

III. The ECT treatment record form

(Prepared by T. Lock)

ECT lends itself to audit and, on the basis of Pippard's findings (1992), is in urgent need of audit in most centres.

This form has been designed with two somewhat conflicting needs in mind: (i) everyday practice and (ii) audit.

For everyday practice, a form should be 'user-friendly', that is, easy to complete by the trainees to whom the task is usually delegated. The more complicated a form, the less likely it is to be completed. On the other hand, the danger of over-simplification is loss of relevant detail (for audit purposes). Furthermore, again with audit in mind, information should be recorded in a manner which facilitates data entry onto a computerised database.

Local clinics are advised to adapt the form, where appropriate, to meet local needs.

PATIENT INFORMATION

Name: _____

Hospital Number: _____

Date of birth: _____

Male/female: _____

Age: _____

In-patient/out-patient: _____

RMO: _____

DIAGNOSIS (Tick several responses if appropriate)

(1) Depression – unipolar ☐ bipolar ☐

(6) Puerperal psychosis ☐

(2) Schizophrenia – type 1 ☐ type 2 ☐ with marked depressive features ☐

(7) Catatonia ☐

(3) Hypomania ☐ mania ☐

(8) Delusional disorder ☐

(4) Mixed affective ☐

(9) Other (specify)

(5) Schizoaffective - depressed ☐ manic ☐

_____

INDICATION FOR ECT: (Tick box if Yes and specify where necessary)

☐ Emergency life-saving procedure
☐ First choice treatment: (specify)
☐ Failed drug treatment: (specify drugs, dose and duration)
☐ Last resort/other: (specify)

CURRENT MEDICATION: (Specify drug, dose, when commenced)

1 _____   5 _____

2 _____   6 _____

3 _____   7 _____

4 _____   8 _____

!!Please discontinue benzodiazepines and carbamazepine if possible!!

Allergies: _____

Recently discontinued medication/substances: (Specify drug, dose, when discontinued)

1 _____   2 _____

RMO's ECT PRESCRIPTION: (Tick correct response)

Bilateral ☐   R. unilateral ☐   L . unilateral ☐

Comments: _____

_____

LEGAL STATUS AT OUTSET: (Tick appropriate box)

1 Informal and consenting, consent form signed   ☐
2 Informal, not consenting, emergency treatment   ☐
3 Detained under Section _____, consenting; consent form signed   ☐
4 Detained under Section _____, not consenting, second opinion   ☐
5 Detained under Section _____, unable to consent, second opinion ☐
6 Detained under Section _____, emergency treatment   ☐

If detained: Is relevant MHA documentation complete and in casenotes?   Yes ☐ No ☐

If second opinion sought: Number of treatments approved _____

LEGAL STATUS AT COMPLETION: (Tick correct response)

Has legal status changed during treatment?
No ☐ Yes ☐ Date of change: _____

If relevant, is MHA documentation complete and in casenotes?   Yes ☐ No ☐

Legal category now (as above): 1 ☐   2 ☐   3 ☐   4 ☐   5 ☐   6 ☐

SYMPTOMS: (Rate 0 if none, 1 if mild, 2 if moderate, 3 if severe; put ratings in box)

Day before first treatment

☐ Concentration difficulties

☐ Memory difficulties

☐ Psychotic delusions

☐ Subjective distress

☐ Endogenous symptoms

Day after last treatment

☐ Concentration difficulties

☐ Memory difficulties

☐ Psychotic delusions

☐ Subjective distress

☐ Endogenous symptoms

PHYSICAL/ANAESTHETIC ASSESSMENT

Date: _____ Pulse: _____ BP: _____ Temperature: _____

PAST/PRESENT MEDICAL AND SURGICAL HISTORY (including gas):

Recent alcohol/drug abuse? No ☐ Yes ☐ (Specify) _____

Smoker? Yes ☐ No ☐

Could patient be pregnant? NA ☐ No ☐ Yes ☐

PHYSICAL EXAMINATION:

CVS:

Respiratory:

CNS:

Abdomen:

Teeth:

INVESTIGATIONS:

NORMAL: ABNORMAL:
Date   Test   Date   Test

‼HAS ANAESTHETIST BEEN INFORMED OF ABNORMALITIES? Yes ☐ No ☐
ANAESTHETIST'S COMMENTS:

PREVIOUS ECT:

Has patient received ECT before? No ☐ Yes ☐ (If Yes, answer below)

1 ☐   2 ☐   3 ☐   4 ☐   5 ☐   6–10 ☐   More ☐ courses of ECT

Clinical response to previous courses (specify): _____

_____

_____

_____

_____

_____

_____

FACTORS THAT RAISE SEIZURE THRESHOLD OR LOWER SEIZURE DURATION
(Tick if Yes)

☐ Over 65   ☐ Benzodiazepines (now or in the last month)
☐ Male   ☐ Carbamazepine (now or in the last month)
☐ Baldness   ☐ Other anticonvulsants
☐ ECT in the last month   ☐ Beta blockers
                             ☐ L-tryptophan

**HAS TRAINEE GIVING FIRST TREATMENT BEEN INFORMED IF ONE OR MORE
POSITIVE RESPONSES TO ABOVE?** Yes ☐ No ☐

DATE:	SESSION 1	SESSION 2
Anaesthetic agent, dose: Muscle relaxant, dose:		
Comments:		
Complications:		
Anaesthetist's signature:		
Stimulation #1 Electrode placement: Dose setting/dose delivered: Impedance test: Seizure pattern: Seizure duration (secs): EEG seizure duration:		
Stimulation #2 Dose setting/dose delivered: Impedance test: Seizure pattern: Seizure duration (secs): EEG seizure duration:		
Stimulation #3 Dose setting/dose delivered: Impedance test: Seizure pattern: Seizure duration (secs): EEG seizure duration:		
Plan for next session:		
Post-ECT side-effects:		

Psychiatrist's signature: _____

RMO comments:

CLINICAL OUTCOME
PATIENT:

		Time after completing ECT			
		1 week	1 month	3 months	6 months
How do you feel compared with how you felt before ECT?	Worse				
	No change				
	Bit better				
	Much better				
	100% well				
What is your memory like now compared with before ECT?	Much worse				
	Bit worse				
	No change				
	Better				

RMO/DEPUTY:

		Time after completing ECT			
		1 week	1 month	3 months	6 months
Global clinical response	Worse				
	No change				
	Improved				
	Full recovery				
Cognitive function outcome	Worse				
	No change				
	Improved				

IV. Consent form

CONSENT

Part A: Patient's consent

I . . . . of . . . .
hereby consent to undergo the administration of a course of ECT (electroconvulsive therapy), the nature, purpose and likely effects of which have been explained to me by

Dr . . . .

I also consent to the administration of an anaesthetic and/or a relaxant or sedative for this purpose.

I understand that an assurance has not been given that the treatment will be administered by a specific practitioner.

Date . . . . Signed . . . .

Part B: Doctor's explanation

I confirm that I have explained to the patient the nature, purpose and likely effect of this treatment.

Date . . . . Signed . . . .

Part C: Record of discussion with relative (where appropriate)

I . . . . of . . . .
and being the . . . . (state nature of relationship)
of . . . . (patient's name) confirm
that an explanation of the nature, purpose and likely effects of ECT (electroconvulsive therapy) has been given to me by Dr . . . . and that I approve of the
treatment being given to my . . . .

Note: Remember that except in the case of a minor, no relative can give consent. While it is recommended that there shall be a relative's approval, the patient shall always be consulted about this first.

Part D: MHA patient
Please tick as appropriate.

  (a) Patient consented, form 38 completed ☐

  (b) Patient unable to consent, form 39 completed ☐

  (c) Patient unable to consent, emergency treatment required ☐

Date .Doctor's signature . . . .

V. Nursing guidelines for ECT

S. M. Halsall, T. Lock & A. Atkinson

The Royal College of Nursing (RCN) prepared guidelines relating to issues specific to nursing practice in ECT clinics in 1982, which were published in the first edition of *The Practical Administration of Electroconvulsive Therapy* (Royal College of Psychiatrists, 1989). The standard of nursing care in ECT clinics improved quite dramatically over the decade separating the two Royal College of Psychiatrists' ECT audits (Pippard & Ellam, 1981; Pippard, 1992).

Nurses working in ECT clinics need to be aware that the Special Committee on ECT of the Royal College of Psychiatrists offers revision courses for consultant psychiatrists and anaesthetists responsible for administering ECT, and have produced a training video *(Electroconvulsive Therapy: The Official Training Video of the Royal College of Psychiatrists, 1994)* with the aim of updating and improving the national standard of ECT practice. Particular attention has focused on the 'technical' aspects of ECT administration (e.g. the optimal use of existing and new models of ECT machines; the selection of an appropriate 'dose' of electricity for a given patient; the correct method of applying the stimulus electrodes) and seizure monitoring. These aspects of ECT have been – *and will remain* – the responsibility of psychiatrists but, because of the multidisciplinary nature of treatment, updating psychiatric practice will have a 'knock-on' effect on all other disciplines working in ECT clinics, and nurses also will be required to update their existing practices and procedures.

These guidelines have been approved by the United Kingdom Central Council for Nursing, Midwifery and Health Visiting (UKCC).

The principles of the nurse's role in ECT are:

(1) ensuring that the psychological needs of patients and statutory requirements are met;
(2) monitoring the patient's physical well-being;
(3) assisting and supporting medical staff in the use of equipment;
(4) supporting and educating patients, relatives and significant others;
(5) supporting, guiding and educating all grades of nursing staff so as to facilitate improvements in ECT practice.

General issues

ECT should be administered in a purpose-built clinic within a hospital, with one trained nurse having overall management responsibility for the ECT clinic. Ideally, the ECT clinic nurse manager should be present at every treatment session. A nominated (and suitably experienced) deputy should take over in his/her absence (e.g. when the clinic manager is on annual leave).

The three stages of treatment comprise patient preparation, administration of treatment, and recovery. A trained nurse should be present at each stage, and each stage should be carried out in physically separate environments. ECT clinics should ideally have a 'core team' of dedicated and experienced nurses who work in the clinic on a regular basis, as this aids continuity of care. It is advisable to use nursing assistants to assist the trained nurses with low skill tasks such as linen changing, patient refreshments, and so on.

In hospitals where ECT is administered in various locations, a coordinating group should be established to ensure a standardised approach to the procedure, and each area should have a nurse nominated to be responsible for the nursing contribution to the procedure. Nurses in charge of ECT clinics in Trusts where ECT is administered in different clinics may also wish to consider establishing a coordinating group.

The ECT nursing team should at all times be aware of their professional abilities and limitations, and each registered nurse member of that team should comply with the requirements of the UKCC's Code of Professional Conduct and the principles for practice set out in other documents from the same source.

Role of the ECT clinic nurse manager

The ECT clinic nurse manager should be a registered first level nurse with experience of ECT practice. Previous general nursing experience is useful.

The manager's main responsibility is to develop the clinic nursing policy and ensure that the policy is adhered to. The nursing policy should be regularly evaluated for its effectiveness. The manager is also responsible for establishing a suitably qualified and committed team of ECT clinic nurses, and for ensuring continuity of care. Maintaining a high standard of nursing care is dependent on active encouragement of a positive attitude to treatment, and support of all grades of clinic nurse. Regular in-service educational programmes (e.g. CPR training, care of the unconscious patient, training in 'new' techniques) should be facilitated and organised.

It is the manager's responsibility to ensure that all necessary equipment meets health and safety recommendations and, where relevant, has been serviced in accordance with the manufacturer's instructions. Equipment should be ready for use and accessible on clinic days. Necessary drugs should be available, and care should be taken to ensure that drugs are not time-expired. There should be a reliable system of re-ordering frequently used items, and spare supplies should be available and accessible. Other clinic nurses should be familiar with the re-ordering procedure.

The manager also has a coordinating role and would be expected to liaise with other ECT clinic professionals, ward managers and ward staff, the patient's responsible medical officer, managers with responsibility for Mental Health Act legislation, community nurses, social workers, relatives and escorts.

Composition of the ECT clinic nursing team

The total number of nurses – and the skill mix of those nurses – who should be present in the ECT clinic on any given treatment day should depend on the number and needs of patients undergoing treatment, not on which nurses happen to be available. Several factors need to be considered: continuity of care, patient safety and patient comfort.

The 'core team'

In forming the core team of dedicated and experienced nurses who work in the clinic on a regular basis, it should be assumed that, while one patient is waiting to be treated, another will be receiving treatment and two more will be in various stages of recovery at any one time. A trained first or second level nurse should supervise each of the three stages (patient preparation, treatment and recovery). As patient preparation precedes treatment, one trained nurse (e.g. the ECT clinic manager) could assume dual responsibility for both these stages. In terms of grading and absolute numbers, the core team should comprise a minimum of one first level nurse (for preparation/treatment) and one further first or second level (enrolled) nurse (for recovery), supported by two further second level (enrolled) nurses or health care assistants. Health care assistants must be trained in specific ECT clinic support duties and must be able to perform these duties competently, before being counted in the core team establishment. The only occasion on which one trained nurse is adequate is when only one patient is scheduled for treatment.

Escort nurses

A nurse known to each patient – ideally the patient's named nurse – should accompany the patient throughout the various stages of treatment. The role of this nurse is to act as the patient's advocate, offering support and reassurance, ensuring that the patient's privacy and dignity is safeguarded, and relaying the patient's anxieties to the core nursing team or medical staff as appropriate. The accompanying nurse may also be required to assist the more experienced members of nursing staff (e.g. in supporting limbs during the seizure). Nursing assistants and students must have a basic understanding of what treatment entails before being allowed to fulfil this role.

Duties of the nurse in the ECT clinic

Phase 1: patient preparation

The ECT clinic nurse manager has overall responsibility for the preparation stage which, in the case of in-patients, begins in the patient's ward of origin. We use a pre-operative checklist which summarises the relevant preparation items outlined below. Most of the items are best attended to by the in-patient's named nurse. The clinic nurse manager ensures that 'last minute' items – which can only be completed when the patient arrives in the ECT suite – have been attended to.

Particular care should be taken in the case of out-patients, for information given by a patient and relatives or friends may be unreliable, and may differ quite markedly from nursing observations. Where possible, out-patients should be encouraged to report to a ward for nursing observations, or, failing that, to the ECT clinic well before the commencement of clinic activities. Out-patients should be given an indication as to how long their treatment will take, and should be advised that it is desirable for them to be accompanied home by a relative or friend, and inadvisable to return to an empty house alone. Furthermore, they should be advised to avoid alcohol, and not to drive a motor vehicle for the rest of the day. Where an out-patient arrives unaccompanied, it is the responsibility of the clinic nurse manager to ensure that the patient is not allowed to leave until fully recovered, and that in no circumstances should the patient be allowed to drive himself home.

Physical

The nurse should ensure that each patient has been examined by the responsible doctor; that physical findings and relevant investigations are available for the anaesthetist; and that the patient has fasted for 6–8 hours in accordance with clinic anaesthetic policy. A record should be available of the patient's pulse, temperature and blood pressure. The patient's medication chart and casenotes should also be made available. The nurse should inform medical staff if the patient has taken any prescribed, legal, or illicit medication or substance which may result in adverse reactions.

Patients should wear loose clothes and an identification bracelet. Patients who normally wear contact lenses should be advised to wear spectacles on treatment days instead. Patients should not be wearing excess make-up or jewellery. Hair clips, valuables, dentures and prostheses should be removed and stored in a safe place, but it is not advisable to remove spectacles and hearing aids before the patient is in the treatment room, as premature removal of such items may result in severe communication difficulties and increased levels of confusion and distress. Patients should be given the opportunity to void urine before the administration of the anaesthetic.

Patients should arrive in the ECT suite at an appointed time so as to facilitate efficient use of clinic resources. Where ECT suites are situated in close proximity to the patient's ward, times of arrival could be staggered so as to avoid lengthy periods of waiting and a congested clinic waiting room.

Psychological

A nurse known to, and trusted by, the patient should escort the patient to the ECT suite and should remain with the patient at least until treatment is administered, and preferably during all the stages of treatment. In the case of in-patients, the ideal escort is the patient's named nurse, while in the case of out-patients, the patient's community nurse or key-worker, or a member of the out-patient department, should perform a similar function. Some agitated patients benefit greatly from the emotional support offered by a relative or friend. In some clinics, informed and cooperative relatives/friends are allowed to accompany patients during all the stages of treatment if both are agreeable, and if clinic staff consider that the patient will benefit.

The nurse should ensure that each patient has been given a full explanation of the nature of the treatment, that the explanation has been understood, and that consenting patients have signed consent to treatment. The nurse should inform medical staff without delay if any patient refuses or is reluctant to accept treatment. It is particularly important to inform medical staff if a patient expresses a desire to withdraw consent.

The likelihood and management of minor side-effects (e.g. a short period of confusion and disorientation immediately after treatment, a headache, and short-term memory problems) should be explained. The nurse should confidently and promptly answer the patient's questions, although certain questions (e.g. medical diagnosis, queries about the anaesthetic, issues relating to the Mental Health Act) are best referred to the appropriate member of the ECT clinic staff. The nurse should remind the patient that he/she will not be left alone, and that qualified doctors and nurses will be in the clinic throughout treatment. Some patients may be confused and disorientated in the immediate recovery stage, and may need considerable reassurance until fully recovered.

Phase 2: administration of treatment

Preparation of the treatment area

Trolleys should be prepared in accordance with clinic policy. An adequate supply of required anaesthetic agents and drugs should be available and accessible. The treatment area nurse should ensure that all safety and treatment equipment is in working order and switched on, and that a spare (full) oxygen cylinder is available. In clinics using ECT machines with built-in EEG monitors, the nurse should ensure that there is an adequate supply of recording paper in the machine, and an accessible spare roll of recording paper. Some ECT machine manufacturers recommend that the stimulus electrodes should be soaked in an electrolyte solution, while others recommend using electrolyte gel or paste. It may be necessary to prepare an electrolyte solution in the first case; alternatively, an adequate supply of electrode paste or gel should be available.

Patient preparation

The treatment area nurse should ensure that 'last minute' patient preparation items have been attended to (e.g. that the patient has voided urine, and that spectacles and hearing aids are removed), and that the patient is comfortably and safely positioned on the trolley. The patient's scalp should be thoroughly cleaned in preparation for application of the stimulus electrodes, and, where EEG monitoring is in use, EEG electrodes. Attention of medical staff should be drawn to any suspected problems or difficulties.

Induction of general anaesthesia

Under no circumstances should the nurse mix, draw up, or administer intravenous anaesthetic agents, as this is the responsibility of the anaesthetist. The nurse should reassure the patient during the induction of anaesthesia.

Hamilton cuff technique

The correct use of this technique is dependent on collaboration between the treatment nurse, the anaesthetist and the treating psychiatrist. A blood pressure cuff is applied to the other arm than that which the anaesthetist intends to use (in the case of right unilateral ECT, the anaesthetist should use the left arm and the cuff should be applied to the right arm). The arterial supply to the arm should be completely occluded by inflating the cuff to about 25 mm mercury above systolic pressure just before the anaesthetist administers the intravenous bolus, and the pressure in the cuff must be maintained until the patient has had an adequate generalised seizure. It is important to ensure that the pressure in the cuff has been released before the patient is wheeled into the recovery area.

Electrical stimulation of the patient

The treating psychiatrist is responsible for the electrical stimulation of patients. The technique used to induce seizures in most clinics is, however, in need of considerable improvement (Pippard, 1992), and updating psychiatric practice is dependent on the cooperation of clinic nurses.

(1) Clinics are being encouraged to update their ECT machines, and nurses will be expected to familiarise themselves with more powerful and sophisticated ECT machines.
(2) Psychiatrists are being encouraged to be more selective with respect to the 'dose' of electricity used to stimulate individual patients. There are several approaches to the problem of 'individualising' the dose of the stimulus, and some trial and error is to be expected in the early stages as clinics develop their 'dosing policy'.
(3) Psychiatrists are also being encouraged to pay particular attention to the way in which they apply the stimulus electrodes to the scalp; to the process of verifying that good electrical contact has been established; and to maintaining good electrical contact until the patient has an adequate generalised seizure.

It is recommended that a trained nurse triggers the electrical stimulus and test function from the ECT machine itself, rather than using the remote button on the stimulus electrodes, for a number of reasons: (a) patient safety (see Appendix VI for comments); (b) to enable the treating psychiatrist to concentrate on establishing and maintaining contact between the electrodes and the scalp. Even the most experienced operators 'wobble' the electrodes when applying pressure to the remote button, which may result in poor contact, skin burns and inadequate stimulation.

What is needed is cooperation similar to that which exists in an operating theatre between a nurse and a surgeon. While the psychiatrist concentrates on maintaining the position of the electrodes, the treatment nurse should alter the relevant switch or dial settings, and press the relevant buttons on the ECT machine, under the verbal direction of the psychiatrist. *It is important that the psychiatrist gives timely sequential instructions to the nurse which can be clearly heard by all the personnel in the treatment room and that the nurse repeats the instructions back to the psychiatrist. Under no circumstances should the nurse make decisions, in particular with respect to the setting of the dial which controls the 'dose' of electricity administered to the patient.* NB: If either the psychiatrist or the nurse is not used to cooperating in this way, a few role-play practice sessions are advisable before undertaking real treatment!

Seizure monitoring

The treating psychiatrist is responsible for ensuring that an adequate seizure has been induced, and for documenting the presence and duration of seizure activity. It may be policy in some clinics to delegate the task of timing the seizures to an experienced nurse.

Some ECT machines have built-in EEG monitoring facilities. The role of the nurse with respect to EEG monitoring is unclear, as few British psychiatrists have experience of EEG monitoring, and very few clinics are equipped with these machines. Additional training will be required for all staff working in clinics equipped with these machines.

Care of the convulsing patient

In most cases it is not necessary or acceptable to apply a strong counter-force during the procedure to restrain the patient, and it is quite safe to allow the limbs to move freely during the tonic and clonic phases of the seizure. Only occasionally, when seizure activity is unusually brisk, will one or more limbs require support and/or gentle restriction. When the Hamilton cuff technique is used, it is important to pay attention to the arm with the pressure cuff, for seizure activity in this arm is likely to be more brisk than in the other limbs. Upon cessation of the seizure, the nurse (or nurses) should replace the limbs in their natural positions.

Immediate post-operative care
The treatment nurse may be required to assist the anaesthetist in the immediate post-operative phase while the patient is still in the treatment room by carrying out some of the tasks which are defined in the following section.

Phase 3: recovery

Responsibility for this phase should be with a trained nurse who is competent in recovery techniques and procedures. Skills should be regularly practised and revised. It is important to ensure that all emergency equipment (e.g. defibrillator, ECG monitor, oral suction) is switched on and ready for use, and recovery nurses should be trained in the use of this equipment. Prompt medical assistance should be accessible for all patients in the recovery phase. Liaison should be maintained with treatment room staff, who should advise the recovery room nurses beforehand of the pending arrival of patients, and whether problems have been encountered in the immediate post-operative phase.

As with all patients recovering from a general anaesthetic, the nurse should ensure that patients are placed in the three-quarter prone recovery position and that a clear airway is maintained. The nurse may be required to carry out oral suction. A nurse should remain with the patient throughout the recovery phase. Pulse, respiration, blood pressure and colour should be monitored at regular intervals. The patient's level of consciousness should be monitored by means of the eyelash reflex and response to verbal commands. Any abnormal observations should be recorded in the nursing notes. It is important to document the duration of confusion and disorientation, if present.

It is important not to rush patients in the recovery phase. Some patients – in particular the elderly – take longer than others to recover fully. Reassurance and support should be on offer for all patients, in particular the unfortunate few whose recovery is complicated by pronounced confusion and disorientation.

Patients who have fully recovered consciousness and who are maintaining their own airway, responsive to verbal commands and willing to move, should be escorted to a quiet and comfortable post-recovery area where they can sit quietly and partake of refreshments. If the ECT suite is situated close to the patient's ward, the patient could be escorted back to the ward instead, provided that the patient is allowed a similar period of peace and quiet to recover fully.

Some patients fail to inform nursing or medical staff of post-operative side-effects such as headache. It is important, therefore, to ask for adverse reactions to treatment. A post-operative checklist (page 121) prompts nurses to ask for the presence or absence of common or worrying side-effects at regular intervals after treatment.

Particular attention should be paid to out-patients, who should not be allowed to return home until they have fully recovered from the 'hangover' effects of the general anaesthetic. Ideally, out-patients should be accompanied home by a friend or relative and in no circumstances should they be allowed to drive themselves home in a motor vehicle.

References

PIPPARD, J. (1992) Audit of electroconvulsive treatment in two National Health Service regions. *British Journal of Psychiatry*, **160**, 621–637.
—— & ELLAM, L. (1981) Electroconvulsive therapy in Great Britain. *British Journal of Psychiatry*, **139**, 563–568.
ROYAL COLLEGE OF PSYCHIATRISTS (1989) *The Practical Administration of Electroconvulsive Therapy*. London: Gaskell.

Nursing checklist for ECT patients

Ward nurse to complete items 1–12 by ✓, X, R (refused) or N/A (not applicable). ECT nurse to re-check and attend to items 13–17.

Patient ID
Weight . . . . kg   Urine test
Could patient be pregnant? Yes/No/NA   Abnormalities
Does patient have/wear: (please specify)
    Dentures   Yes/No
    Capped teeth   Yes/No
    Hearing aid   Yes/No
    Spectacles   Yes/No

Ward . . . . or out-patient . . . .

Session	1	2	3	4	5	6	7	8	9
1) Correct patient (fit ID label or nameband)									
2) Correct casenotes & prescription record									
3) ECT record complete & in casenotes									
4) ECT clinic nurse informed of any abnormalities? (page 3, ECT record)									
5) (a) Consent form in ECT pack OR (b) MHA documentation in casenotes									
6) Relevant investigation results in casenotes (CXR, ECG, bloods)									
7) (a) Blood pressure (b) Pulse (c) Temperature									
8) When did patient last pass urine (time)?									
9) When did patient last eat or drink?									
10) Has makeup been removed?									
11) Hair shampooed night before and not wearing hair lacquer, gel, etc.?									
12) Jewellery & hair pins removed?									
13)* Anaesthetist informed of any abnormalities?									
14)* Artificial eyes/contact lenses removed?									
15)* Electrode sites prepared?									
16)* Dentures removed?									
17)* Hearing aid/spectacles removed?									
COMMENTS									
Signature (ward nurse)									
Signature (ECT nurse)									

ECT post-operative nursing observations

Date:

Treatment session:

Time	Before ECT	10 mins	30 mins	1 hour	3 hours	6 hours
Temperature						
Blood pressure						
Pulse						
Respiration						
Routine questions (please tick or cross) 1) What is your first name? 2) What is your last name? 3) How old are you? 4) What year were you born? 5) What country do we live in? 6) What city do we live in? 7) What is the name of this hospital? 8) What year is it now? 9) What month is it? 10) What day is it today?						
(Yes or no) Do you have a headache? Do you feel like being sick/wanting to vomit? Do your muscles feel sore?						
Is patient agitated?						
Have you reported any abnormalities to nursing staff?						
Has the medical officer been informed of any difficulties?						

VI. Review of ECT machines

T. Lock

Selecting an ECT machine is not an easy matter, and a thorough understanding of the equipment is essential if it is to be used competently. Machines differ with respect to the characteristics of the stimulus generated, the means of controlling that stimulus, and other features that may be built in. Some of these are important for safety reasons; some are useful but not essential; and others offer little if any practical advantage, despite claims to the contrary by the manufacturers. The 'best buy' for local use requires a general understanding of the merits and limitations of available equipment, and of local ECT practice.

We have reviewed machines manufactured by two British Companies (Ectron Limited and Sycopel Scientific Limited) and two American Companies (Mecta Corporation and Somatics Incorporated). The Siemens Konvulsator (a model used widely in Europe and Scandinavia), Medcraft and Elcot machines (both manufactured in the US) have not been included, as they are not readily available in Britain. For further information on Ectron machines, see Russell (1988). Stephens *et al* (1991) provide a good review of American ECT machines. Front panel diagrams are given in in this section. Tables 3 and 4 provide a comparative summary of technical and other characteristics.

No single machine is ideal; all have some drawbacks. We have ranked acceptable equipment on seven criteria (see below) to arrive at a short list of four models – 'British version' Mecta SR2 and JR2, Thymatron-DGx and Ectron Series 5A Ectonus machines – which we think are suitable for routine NHS clinical work.

Machines manufactured by Ectron Limited, UK

Sales and maintenance: Ectron Limited, Knap Close, Letchworth, Herts SG6 1AQ
Telephone 01462 682124
Fax 01462 481463

Ectron Limited has manufactured and supplied ECT machines since 1939, and has been the main – or only – British manufacturer for over 20 years. Prior to 1973 machines generated a sine-wave stimulus, and from 1973 to 1982 a chopped sine-wave stimulus. Constant current brief-pulse equipment was introduced in 1981. Four generations of brief-pulse ECT machines were produced between 1981 and 1993: Series 1, Series 2, Series 3 and Series 5. Clinics in the south of England were equipped almost exclusively with Ectron machines in 1992 (Pippard, 1992): Series 5 (54%), Series 2 and 3 (37%) and earlier models (9%). All of these models must now be considered obsolete. The company introduced their latest machine, the Series 5A, in 1993.

The manufacturer provides a reliable and easily accessible after-sales service.

ECTRON SERIES 5A ECTONUS AND ECTONUSTIM

Year of manufacture: July 1993 onwards
Price at June 1994: £2700 (Ectonus); £2900 (Ectonustim)
Dimensions: 30.5 cm × 16 cm × 19 cm; approx. 4.6 kg; metal casing (prototypes were in a light oak casing)

Table 3. How general and safety features of ECT machines compare with the "ideal" (as of 1 August 1994)

Model	Waveform	Output control	Test function	Auto stimulus abort	Audible signal	Visual signal	Output display (mC)	Print-out	Dual EEG	Suitable electrodes	Mains supply	Used by
"Ideal"	**b BP**	**1**	**Y**	**Y**	**Y**	**Y**	**Y**	**+**	**+**	**Y**	**D**	
ECTRON (UK)												
Mark 4	u/b csin	1	N	N	Y	Y	N	N	N	Y	D	obs
Series 2/3	u BP	2	N	N	Y	Y	N	N	N	Y	D	obs
Series 2+/3+[1]	u BP	2	N	N	Y	Y	N	N	N	Y	D	obs
Series 5	u BP	1	Y	N	Y	Y	Y	N	N	Y	D	mc
Series 5A	u BP	1	Y	N	Y	Y	Y	N	N	Y	D	S
NEUROTRONIC (UK)												
Research	u/b BP	5	N	N	Y	N	N	N	N	Y	D	F
Standard	b BP	1	N	N	Y	N	N	N	N	Y	D	-
MECTA (US)												
JR2i (Brit)	b BP	1	Y	Y	Y	Y	Y	N	N	Y	D	-
SR2 (Brit)	b BP	1	Y	Y	Y	Y	Y	Y	Y	Y	T	L; S
JR1 (Brit)	b BP	4	Y	Y	Y	Y	Y	N	N	Y	T	-
SR1 (Brit)	b BP	4	Y	Y	Y	Y	Y	Y	Y	Y	T	-
JR2i (IEC)	b BP	1	Y	Y	Y	Y	Y	N	N	Y	D	-
SR2 (IEC)	b BP	1	Y	Y	Y	Y	Y	Y	Y	Y	T	-
JR1 (IEC)	b BP	4	Y	Y	Y	Y	Y	N	N	Y	T	-
SR1 (IEC)	b BP	4	Y	Y	Y	Y	Y	Y	Y	Y	T	-
JR2 (US)	b BP	1	Y	Y	Y	Y	Y	N	N	Y	D	-
SR2 (US)	b BP	1	Y	Y	Y	Y	Y	Y	Y	Y	T	-
JR1(US)	b BP	4	Y	Y	Y	Y	Y	N	N	Y	T	-
SR1 (US)	b BP	4	Y	Y	Y	Y	Y	Y	Y	Y	T	-
SOMATICS												
Thymatron DGx	b BP	1/3	Y	Y	Y	Y	Y	Y	Y	Y	D	B; L
Thy. DGx (-mon)[2]	b BP	1	Y	Y	Y	Y	Y	N	N	Y	D	-

1. Modified Ectron Series 2/Series 3.
2. Thymatron DGx without graph/printer.
Output control (1 to 5) = number of dials/switches which the operator must set for a given charge output. For Thymatron DGx, output is controlled by one dial in 'standard' and FlexiDial 'Energy x 2' modes; 3 dials in unmodified FlexiDial mode.
BP, brief pulse, constant current; csin, 60% chopped sine wave; u, uniphasic; b, biphasic; Y or N, model does or does not incorporate a feature considered essential; +, feature regarded as advantageous but not essential; D, connects directly to British mains; T, connects to a transformer; obs, obsolete; mc, manufacture ceased.
Used by ECT Committee member in charge of a local clinic: B, Benbow; F, Fergusson; L, Lock; S, Scott.

Table 4. How technical features of ECT machines compare with the "ideal" (as of 1 August 1994)

Model	Minimum output charge (mC)	Maximum output charge (mC)	Minimum stimulus intensity (mC/s)	Maximum stimulus intensity (mC/s)	Output increments (mC)	Minimum current (mA)	Maximum current (mA)	Minimum stimulus duration (s)	Maximum stimulus duration (s)	Minimum pulse width (ms)	Maximum pulse width (ms)	Minimum frequency (Hz)	Maximum frequency (Hz)	Maximum voltage output (V)	Maximum impedance for c.c. (Ω)	Ease of modification	BS compatibility
"Ideal"	25	>1000	?	?	25–50	?	1000	2	6	1	?	?	<90	?	?	Y	Y
Mark 4[1] (2)	162	inf.	95	—	—		760	1.7	inf.	2.5	2.5	50	50	198	n/a	N	Y
(4)	44	255	9				1060	5	5	0.33	0.33	25	25	318			
Series 2/3	28	350	28	43	28/42	850	850	1	6	1.25	1.25	26	40	225	450	N	Y
Series 2+/3+	37	400	37	58	37/58	850	850	1	6	1.25	1.25	35	55	225	450	N	Y
Series 5	150	400	46	123	25	750	750	3.25	3.25	2.2	2.2	28	74	225	500	N	Y
Series 5A	50	700	50	116	var	750	750	1	6	2.2	2.2	30	70	225	500	N	Y
Research	7.5	4455	25	743	var	100	990	1	6	1.5	2.5	50	150			N	Y
Standard	120	780	40	260	6	200	1200	3	3	1	1	100	100			N	Y
JR2i (Brit)	25	1200	44	202	25/50	550	800	0.5	5.96	1	1.4	40	90	240	400	Y	Y
SR2 (Brit)	25	1200	44	202	25/50	550	800	0.5	5.96	1	1.4	40	90	240	400	Y	Y
JR1 (Brit)	22	1152	44	288	var	550	800	0.5	4	1	2	40	90	240	400	Y	Y
SR1 (Brit)	22	1152	44	288	var	550	800	0.5	4	1	2	40	90	240	400	Y	Y

Table 4 cont.

Model	Minimum output charge (mC)	Maximum output charge (mC)	Minimum stimulus intensity (mC/s)	Maximum stimulus intensity (mC/s)	Output increments (mC)	Minimum current (mA)	Maximum current (mA)	Minimum stimulus duration (s)	Maximum stimulus duration (s)	Minimum pulse width (ms)	Maximum pulse width (ms)	Minimum frequency (Hz)	Maximum frequency (Hz)	Maximum voltage output (V)	Maximum impedance for c.c. (Ω)	Ease of modification	BS compatibility
JR2i (IEC)	22.4	403.2	140	144	1.48	800	800	0.16	2.8	1	1	90	90	240	400	Y	Y
SR2 (IEC)	22.4	403.2	140	144	1.48	800	800	0.16	2.8	1	1	90	90	240	400	Y	Y
JR1 (IEC)	22	403.2	44	202	var	550	800	0.5	2	1	1.4	40	90	240	400	Y	Y
SR1 (IEC)	22	403.2	44	202	var	550	800	0.5	2	1	1.4	40	90	240	400	Y	Y
JR2(USA)	22	576	220[4]	144[4]	2.16	800	800	0.1	4	1	1	90	90	240	400	Y	Y
SR2 (USA)	22	576	220[4]	144[4]	2.16	800	800	0.1	4	1	1	90	90	240	400	Y	Y
JR1 (USA)	22	576	44	288	var	550	800	0.50	2	1	2	40	90	240	400	Y	Y
SR1 (USA)	22	576	44	288	var	550	800	0.50	2	1	2	40	90	240	400	Y	Y
ThymatronDGx	25.2	504	53	126	25.2	900	900	0.47	4	1.0	1.0	30	70	450	500	Y	Y
Thy. DGx (FD)[2]	25.2	504	27	189	var	900	900	0.16	8	0.5	1.5	30	70	450	500	Y	Y
Thy. DGx (FDx2)[3]	50.4	1008	186	191	50.4	900	900	0.26	5.3	1.5	1.5	70	70	450	500	Y	Y

1. Mark 4 constant voltage machine: output varies inversely with impedance. Figures assume a 300 Ω impedance; (4) = uniphasic sinewave; (2) = uniphasic ultra brief pulse. Other models constant current (c.c.) machines if impedance is within range.
2. ThymatronDGx connected to FlexiDial.
3. Thymatron DGx in Flexidial 'Energy x 2' mode.
4. Values due to predetermined stimulus duration values at minimum and maximum charge settings.
Pulse width refers to the central section of the sine wave; actual phase width is greater.
var, variable (increment determined by the operator); inf, infinite (determined by operator)
Missing data not supplied by the manufacturers.

Description

These are the latest constant current Ectron models, which are essentially modified versions of the preceding Series 5 models, offering an extended range of stimulus output (50–700 mC, compared with 150–400 mC). The Ectonustim is identical to the Ectonus, but incorporates a 'cerebral stimulator' which delivers a low voltage uniphasic sine-wave stimulus. The manufacturer suggests two uses for the cerebral stimulator: (1) "to give a painful stimulus in conjunction with therapeutic suggestions for the treatment of hysteria" and (2) as a "counter stimulus to reduce amnesia and confusion".

Ectron Series 5 models generate a unique waveform which is said to be particularly effective and associated with fewer cognitive problems. The treatment stimulus is preceded by an 'auto-crescendo' (i.e. build up of stimulus current over a period of 0.25 seconds) which is said to give a gentle onset to the treatment.

Stimulus characteristics

Waveform: Split uniphasic brief-pulse (1.0 ms, 0.6 ms, 0.6 ms) (see Fig. 6, page 90).
Pulse width: Fixed (i.e. non-variable) (combined) pulse width 2.2 ms; phase width 3.4 ms.
Current: Fixed at 750 mA throughout the output range under 50–500 Ω load. Voltage varies with dynamic impedance; maximum voltage 225 V.
Pulse frequency: Automatically varied from 30 to 70 Hz.
Stimulus duration: Automatically varied from 1–6 s (time excludes 0.25 s auto-crescendo).
Output range: 50–700 mC; maximum stimulus intensity 116 mC/s.

Output control

Single dial, calibrated in millicoulombs (mC). Small (approx. 25 mC) dose increments are marked on an inner scale from 1 to 25.

Output display

The stimulus dose actually delivered is displayed on a digital display panel.

Monitoring

Machines do not incorporate ECG or EEG monitoring, and cannot be connected to free standing monitors.

Safety features

The machine has a test function, for static impedance. The passage of stimulus is indicated both audibly and visually. There is no warning given before the passage of current. There is no automatic stimulus abort function. Machines are constructed and certified to BS 5724 Part 1, and IEC 601-1[7].

Input supply

Machines can be connected directly to the British mains (240 V, 60 Hz AC) or to a 110 V, 40 Hz AC supply.

---

7. The administration of a dose in excess of 504 mC is inconsistent with IEC 601-1.

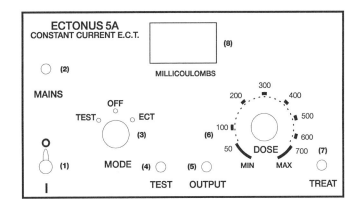

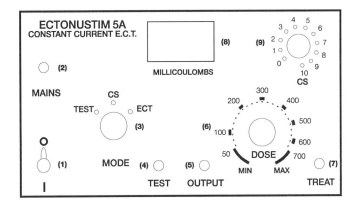

(1)   Mains on/off switch
(2)   Mains on/off indicator light
(3)   Mode switch
(4)   Self-test indicator
(5)   Stimulus indicator light
(6)   Dose output control dial
(7)   Treat button
(8)   Digital display of dose delivered
(9)   Cerebral stimulator dial (on Ectonustim models only)

Other

Hand-held electrodes are suited to the 'traditional' method of establishing patient-to-electrode contact.

Comments

Information supplied by manufacturer

The 'auto-crescendo' function has little if any practical advantage for ECT administered under general anaesthesia. The 'cerebral stimulator' function is redundant. There is no scientific evidence to support the claim that a 'counter stimulus' reduces amnesia or confusion, and the therapeutic use of a non-convulsive painful stimulus amounts to aversive shock therapy – an outdated behaviourist technique sharing nothing in common with ECT.

There is no scientific proof that a split uniphasic pulse is more effective at inducing therapeutic seizures and/or is associated with fewer cognitive side-effects compared with the biphasic waveforms generated by all other machines, or that small dose increments "are useful in a course of treatment, particularly in elderly patients".

No information is provided on threshold titration strategies. Limited stimulus dosing information is available from experience with the Series 5 model. Guidelines for stimulus dosing with the Series 5A are given on page 78.

Other

Upgrading to a Series 5A from an existing Series 5 machine necessitates the purchase of a new machine. The potential for modifications (of predetermined stimulus parameter values) is limited given existing technical constraints and it is unlikely that these machines could be modified to connect to an EEG monitor.

The maximum output may be inadequate for a small number of patients with very high seizure thresholds. The absence of an automatic stimulus abort feature has safety implications and we recommend that the stimulus is triggered from the machine by a trained third party.

The main advantage of the Series 5A model is that practitioners can draw on personal experience of using the preceding Series 5 model. One member of the ECT Committee (Dr Alan Scott) is presently using this machine at the Royal Edinburgh Hospital.

Rankings: (1 = best; 7 = worst)

Safety: 4
Stimulus parameters: 5
Output range: 5
Ease of use: 1
Dose titration: 4
After-sales: 1
Price: 1

ECTRON SERIES 5 ECTONUS AND ECTONUSTIM

Year of manufacture   1987–1993
                           Models have been superseded by Series 5A machines, and are no longer in production
Dimensions   30.5 cm × 16 cm × 19 cm; approx. 4.6 kg; light oak casing

Description

The Ectonustim is identical to the Ectonus, but incorporates a 'cerebral stimulator' (see Series 5A).

Series 5 models offer a narrower range of stimulus output compared to Series 5A models (viz. 150–400 mC, versus 50–700 mC), and stimulus duration is fixed at 3.25 seconds. In other technical respects, Series 5 and Series 5A models are identical.

Compared with earlier models (Series 3 and Series 2 – see below), Series 5 machines generate a more intense stimulus at maximum output setting (123 mC/s versus 58.9 mC/s or 42.8 mC/s for modified and unmodified versions respectively). Maximum charge output (400 mC) compares with 354 mC and 255 mC respectively.

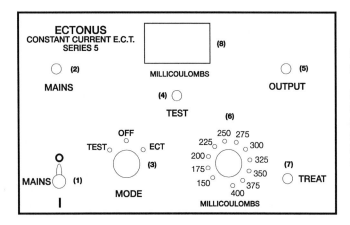

(1)   Mains on/off switch
(2)   Mains on/off indicator light
(3)   Mode switch
(4)   Self-test indicator
(5)   Stimulus indicator light
(6)   Dose output control dial
(7)   Treat button
(8)   Digital display of dose delivered

Comments

See under Series 5A models for comments applicable to the 'auto-crescendo' and 'cerebral stimulator' functions. The narrow range of stimulus output (150–400 mC) does not facilitate dose titration in persons with low seizure thresholds, and the maximum output is insufficient to induce adequate seizures in about 5–10 % of the population. Parts and maintenance will remain available for a period of seven years from date of purchase. Clinics using these models are advised to upgrade their equipment.

ECTRON SERIES 2 ECTONUS AND DUOPULSE, AND SERIES 3 DUOPULSE AND ECTONUSTIM

Year of manufacture	1981–1987
	These models are obsolete
Dimensions	Series 3: 30.5 cm × 15 cm × 18 cm; 3.5. kg; light oak casing
	Series 2: 18 cm × 18 cm × 15 cm; 2.5. kg; mahogany casing with lid; lid contains clips for electrode storage

Description

These are second and third generation constant current brief-pulse Ectron machines. Series 3 models look similar to Series 5 models, while Series 2 models look similar to Mark 4 models (see below).

Series 3 and Series 2 Duopulse models are virtually identical as far as ECT is concerned. The Series 3 Ectonustim is identical to the Duopulse, but incorporates a 'cerebral stimulator'. They generate a uniphasic brief-pulse waveform with a fixed pulse width of 1.25 ms. Current remains constant at 850 mA under a 50–450 Ω load. Duopulse and Ectonustim models offer a total of 12 stimulus output settings, by switching pulse frequency from 26 Hz (ECT 1 setting) to 40 Hz (ECT 2 setting) and by varying stimulus duration from 1–6 seconds.

Some of the earlier Ectonus models offered only one frequency setting and four stimulus duration settings (1–4 s). Ectonus models incorporate an 'Ectonus function', controlled by a semi-rotary 'Ectonus' dial. The 'Ectonus technique' was claimed to give a smooth onset of the tonic stage and control over the clonic stage, thus eliminating the need for muscle relaxant and anaesthetic!

Comments

See under Series 5A for comments relevant to the auto-crescendo and cerebral stimulator functions. It is not clear what the Ectonus technique was, or what the Ectonus dial controlled: in Mark 4 models (see below) the Ectonus dial allowed the operator to override automatic timing of stimulus duration.

Series 3 and Series 2 models manufactured prior to 1985 were underpowered, and the maximum output failed to induce seizures in a sizeable proportion of patients. The manufacturers addressed this problem in 1985, and increased the power output (throughout the output range) by increasing pulse frequency at the ECT 1 and ECT 2 settings from 25 Hz (ECT 1) and 40 Hz (ECT 2) to 35 Hz and 55 Hz respectively. The maximum charge output (354 mC) of modified Series 2 and Series 3 machines (i.e. Series 2+ and Series 3+) compares to 255 mC, and maximum stimulus intensity (58.9 mC/s) compares with 42.5 mC/s of unmodified models. Some Series 3 and Series 2 machines produced before 1985 were returned to the manufacturer for modification, as described above. The increased power output of Series 3+ and Series 2+ machines remained insufficient for effective treatment of all patients.

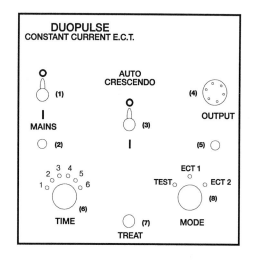

(1)   Mains on/off switch
(2)   Mains on/off indicator light
(3)   Auto-crescendo switch
(4)   Connector for electrodes
(5)   Stimulus indicator light
(6)   Stimulus duration dial
(7)   Treat button
(8)   Mode switch

(1)   Mains on/off switch
(2)   Mains on/off indicator light
(3)   Auto-crescendo switch
(4)   Connector for electrodes
(5)   Stimulus indicator light
(6)   Stimulus duration dial
(7)   Treat button
(8)   Mode switch

(1)   Mains on/off switch
(2)   Mains on/off indicator light
(3)   Auto-crescendo switch
(4)   Connector for electrodes
(5)   Stimulus indicator light
(6)   Self-test indicator
(7)   Treat button
(8)   Mode switch

In 1992 approximately 20% of clinics were still using unmodified Series 3 or Series 2 machines, and 17% were using modified Series 3 or Series 3 machines (Pippard, 1992). These clinics should upgrade their equipment as a matter of urgency.

ECTRON MARK 4 MODELS

Year of manufacture   1969–1982
                             These models are obsolete
Dimensions   21.6 cm × 21.6 cm × 15.3 cm; 4.2 kg; mahogany case with lid for
                             electrode storage

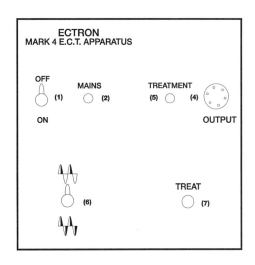

(1)   Mains on/off switch
(2)   Mains on/off indicator light
(4)   Connector for electrodes
(5)   Stimulus indicator light
(6)   Waveform switch (uniphasic
        or biphasic sine wave)
(7)   Treat button
(8)   Ectonus control

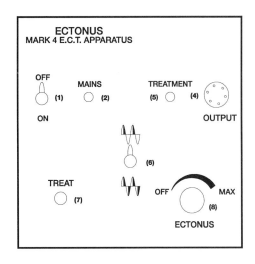

(1)   Mains on/off switch
(2)   Mains on/off indicator light
(4)   Connector for electrodes
(5)   Stimulus indicator light
(6)   Waveform switch (uniphasic
        or biphasic sine wave)
(7)   Treat button
(8)   Ectonus control

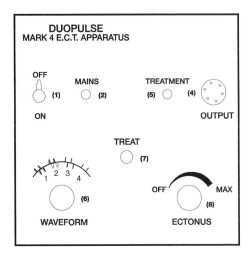

(1)   Mains on/off switch
(2)   Mains on/off indicator light
(4)   Connector for electrodes
(5)   Stimulus indicator light
(6)   Waveform switch (uniphasic
        or biphasic sine wave,
        uniphasic or biphasic ultra
        brief pulse)
(7)   Timer switch for stimulus
        duration

Description

Four different models were produced: Ectron, Ectonus, Ectonustim and Duopulse. All Mark 4 models generate a triangular (60% chopped sine-wave) stimulus, which can be switched from uniphasic to biphasic. Pulse width for uniphasic sine-wave stimulation refers to the central portion of the waveform.

Ectonus models incorporate an 'Ectonus' function controlled by a semi-rotary 'Ectonus' dial, which enables the operator to override automatic timing of stimulus duration. Stimulus duration in uniphasic or biphasic mode is automatically terminated after 1.7 seconds unless the Ectonus function is used. Ectonustim models incorporate a 'cerebral stimulator'. Duopulse models offer a total of four stimulus waveforms: (1) biphasic sine-wave, (2) uniphasic sine-wave, (3) biphasic ultra brief-pulse, and (4) uniphasic ultra brief-pulse (see Fig. 5, page 89). The pulse width of the brief pulse was 0.25 ms and stimulus duration was fixed at 5 seconds. The manufacturer recommended that waveform 1 should be used to treat disturbed psychotic patients, waveform 2 for melancholic states, waveform 3 for less severe depression, and waveform 4 when minimum amnesia and confusion were required.

Mark 4 machines operated on the constant voltage principle, so current, charge and stimulus intensity vary inversely with impedance: e.g. for uniphasic current and stimulus duration of 1.7 s, 225 mC charge is delivered under a 200 Ω load and 95 mC under 300 Ω (400 mC and 162 mC in biphasic mode). The maximum output in uniphasic brief-pulse mode is 44 mC (stimulus duration 5 s), giving a stimulus intensity of 9 mC/s.

Comments

Mark 4 machines (in sine-wave mode) deliver more power, and a higher stimulus intensity, compared with Series 2 and Series 3 brief-pulse models, and are sufficiently powered to induce therapeutic seizures in nearly all patients. Sine-wave stimulation is associated with a greater degree of cognitive side-effects compared with brief-pulse stimulation, and machines generating a sine or chopped sine waveform should no longer be used. Pulse widths of less than 1 ms are ineffective at inducing seizures, and the output of Duopulse machines in either of the brief-pulse modes is not able to induce seizures in all but a few patients. There is no scientific basis for the manufacturer's recommendations with respect to using certain waveforms for certain categories of psychiatric patients and/or symptom severity.

About 9% of clinics in the south of England were still using Mark 4 models in 1992 (Pippard, 1992). These clinics should upgrade their equipment as a matter of urgency.

Machines manufactured by Sycopel Scientific Ltd, UK

Sales and maintenance CR2 6PL   SLE, 232 Selsdon Road, South Croydon, Surrey,

Telephone 0181 681 1414
Fax 0181 649 8570

Neurotronic Therapy System machines are presently in use in a few clinics in the north of England and in Scotland. The original machine – now known as the 'Research' (068-100) model – was designed by the Regional Medical Physics Department, Northern Regional Health Authority, and was manufactured by a local Newcastle electronic company in 1986. A different company, Sycopel Scientific Limited, is now manufacturing these machines. A new model – the 'Standard' (068-200) – was introduced in 1993.

The after-sales service provided by the previous manufacturer of Neurotronic machines was unreliable. The present manufacturer is committed to providing a maintenance service for earlier versions. The reliability of this service is not yet known.

SLE NTS-R (previously NEUROTRONIC 068-100 'RESEARCH' Model)

Year of manufacture   1993 onwards (prototypes manufactured in 1986)
Price at Jan 1995   £3450 (excl. VAT)
Dimensions   47 cm × 33 cm × 11 cm; 9 kg; metal casing

Description

The Research model is a very powerful (maximum output 4455 mC) constant current brief-pulse machine which offers independent control of five brief-pulse stimulus parameters. Its design has been claimed to represent "the first major advance in ECT for 40 years".

Unlike the American machines, this machine is not controlled by a microprocessor. It incorporates a 'soft start function' which is said to minimise cognitive side-effects: The function entails progressively increasing current amplitude from 0 to the selected current value, over a period of 1 second[8]. Its designers have resisted advice to incorporate an impedance test function and a display of the dose actually delivered to the patient on the basis that these functions "are not considered necessary", and maintain that current is the dominant parameter with respect to inducing effective seizures.

Stimulus characteristics

Waveform: Brief-pulse; can be switched from uniphasic to biphasic.
Pulse width: Variable: 1.5, 2, 2.5 ms.
Current: Can be varied from 100 mA to 990 mA with 10 mA increments; constant under a 200 Ω load. Voltage varies with dynamic impedance; maximum voltage output 200 V under a 220 Ω load.
Stimulus duration: Variable; 1–6 seconds (1 second increments).
Pulse frequency: Variable; 50–150 Hz (50 Hz increments).
Output/range: 7.5–4455 mC; Maximum stimulus intensity 742 mC/s.

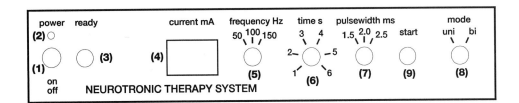

(1)   Mains on/off switch key operated
(2)   Mains on/off indicator
(3)   Indicator ('ready to be used')
(4)   Current output control dial
(5)   Frequency control dial
(6)   Stimulus duration control dial
(7)   Pulse width control dial
(8)   Waveform switch (uniphasic or biphasic brief-pulse stimulation
(9)   Treat button

---

8. 0.25 seconds is quoted in older literature.

Output control

There are four control dials (current, stimulus duration, frequency and pulse width) and one switch (uniphasic/biphasic). Several parameter settings must be selected by the operator to effect a desired output, and the dose (in mC) must be manually calculated or obtained from tables with reference to stimulus parameter settings.

Output display

The machine does not display the dose actually delivered to the patient.

Monitoring

The machines does not incorporate ECG or EEG monitoring, and cannot be connected to free-standing monitors.

Safety features

The machine does not have a self-test function or an automatic stimulus abort function. It indicates the passage of the stimulus audibly but not visibly; a continuous tone is emitted when the machine is able to maintain the selected current value, and a warbling tone is emitted when it is unable to maintain current at the set level due to high impedance values. In such circumstances, the machine automatically repeats the 'soft start' procedure.

The machine is constructed to BS 5724 Part 1 and IEC 601-1.[9]

Input supply

The machine connects directly to British mains (240 V; 60 Hz, AC).

Other

Hand-held electrodes are supplied which are suitable for the recommended method of establishing patient-to-electrode contact.

Comments

Information supplied by the manufacturer
Conflicting technical data (e.g. duration of 'soft start' function) is quoted in the information supplied by the different manufacturers.

Given the design of contemporary American machines, incorporating several safety features which are not included on this model, it is debateable whether the Neurotronic 'Research' machine represents a major advance in ECT machine design. We do not agree that a test for static impedance, and a display of the dose actually delivered to the patient are "not considered necessary".

The 'soft start' function is similar to the 'auto-crescendo' function on Ectron machines, and is of limited value for ECT given under general anaesthesia; there is, furthermore, no evidence that this function reduces cognitive side-effects.

The manufacturers provide little, if any, guidance on stimulus dosing strategies, and do not provide tables for stimulus output (in mC) at different stimulus parameter settings.

---

9. The administration of a dose in excess of 504 mC is inconsistent with IEC 601-1.

Other

The need for, and safety of, the huge maximum output of 4455 mC is questionable. We can see no possible justification for producing a machine which can deliver such large amounts of energy. The machine is complicated to use and therefore carries a higher than average potential for clinical error in inexperienced hands (e.g. inadvertently administering the maximum power output). Competent use of the machine is dependent on a high standard of training and supervision. It is not recommended for routine clinical use, and is best suited to research clinics wishing to study brief-pulse stimulation characteristics. Because there is no automatic stimulus abort function, it is recommended that the stimulus is triggered by a trained third party from the machine itself. It is not known whether modifications of the existing design are possible, and our experience has been that suggestions for modification have been resisted.

The seizure threshold titration strategy is based on the experience of one user[10] who developed the strategy by trial and error and with help from H. Sackeim and R. Weiner in the US. Guidelines for stimulus dosing with this machine are given in Chapter 22, based on experience with this machine at the Doncaster Royal Infirmary and Argyll and Bute Hospital.

There is some evidence to support the claim that current is the dominant parameter with respect to inducing seizures with this model. Users report that seizures are not reliably induced at current strengths less than 550 mA, or output doses of less than 120 mC (current 800 mA, 50 Hz, stimulus duration 1.0 s, pulse width 1.5 ms, biphasic. The reason for high starting doses (see page 80) relative to other machines is unclear, but may be related to the fact that the 'soft start function' reduces the effective stimulus duration.

The original Research machines could be triggered by switches on the machine, the electrodes, and by a foot switch. The foot switch was a useful practical feature, but its use is not permitted under IEC 601-1. It has been omitted from models manufactured after 1993.

One member of the ECT Committee (Dr Grace Fergusson) is presently using a 1986 prototype.

Rankings: (1 = best; 7 = worst)

Safety:	6
Stimulus parameters:	4
Output range:	4
Ease of use:	6
Dose titration:	4
After sales:	?
Price:	2

SLE NTS-C (previously NEUROTRONIC 068-200 STANDARD Model)

Year of manufacture	November 1993 onwards
Price at June 1994	£3300 (excl. VAT)
Dimensions	47 cm × 33 cm × 11 cm; 14 kg; metal casing

Description

This machine is a modified version of the 'Research' (SLE NTS-R) prototype and is considerably simpler to use. It differs from the 'Research' model in that it generates a

---

10. Dr Karel de Pauw, Doncaster Royal Infirmary.

biphasic brief-pulse waveform only, with a fixed pulse width of 1 ms, fixed pulse frequency of 100 Hz and fixed stimulus duration of 3 seconds. Stimulus output (in mC) is therefore under the control of a single dial, which varies current in 10 mA increments from 200 to 1200 mA. Each 10 mA increment corresponds to a charge increment of 6 mC. The range of power output is 120–780 mC. Output tables (in mC) at different current settings are not provided. Like its 'Research' counterpart, the 'Standard' model does not display the charge actually delivered to the patient, and does not possess a test function for static impedance or an automatic stimulus abort function.

Comments

See under 'SLE NTS-R' for comments on the absence of a display panel, self-test and stimulus abort function. The predetermined (fixed) pulse frequency (100 Hz) setting is significantly above the upper limit (83 Hz) for effective neuronal depolarisation/repolarisation. It is not known whether modifications of the existing design are possible, and our experience has been that suggestions for modification have been resisted.

The use of current as the main dose output variable means that output (in mC) must be calculated or obtained with reference to tables (which the practitioner must devise himself/herself). No information is available on stimulus dosing strategies, and no member of the ECT Committee is using one of these machines. The range of stimulus output is relatively narrow and it is likely that the lowest output dose (120 mC) will be too high to enable accurate dose titration in patients with low seizure thresholds, while the maximum dose output (780 mC) may be insufficient for a small number of patients with very high seizure thresholds.

Because there is no automatic stimulus abort function, it is recommended that the stimulus is triggered by a trained third party from the machine itself.

Rankings: (1 = best; 7 = worst)

Safety: 4
Stimulus parameters: 6
Output range: 5
Ease of use: 1
Dose titration: 4
After sales: ?
Price: 5

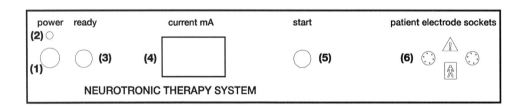

(1)   Mains on/off switch key operated
(2)   Mains on/off indicator
(3)   Indicator ('ready to be used')
(4)   Current output control dial
(5)   Treat button
(6)   Electrode sockets

Machines manufactured by the Mecta Corporation, US

Address   7015 S.W. McKewan Road, Lake Oswego, Oregon 97035, US
Telephone (US) 503 6248778
Fax (US) 503 624 8729

Sales and maintenance   Medelec Vickers Limited
Manor Way, Old Woking, Surrey GU22 9JU
Telephone 01483 770331
Fax 01483 727193

The first commercially available constant current brief-pulse ECG/EEG Monitored Electro-Convulsive Therapy Apparatus (Mecta) was developed at the Oregan Health Sciences Centre in 1973. The original manufacturing company was incorporated into the Mecta Corporation in 1980, and second generation (Series D) Mecta machines were introduced in 1981. The present Mecta SR1, JR1, SR2 and JR2 models were introduced in 1985. The Mecta Corporation began to market their products in Britain in 1992 through the British Medical Instrument Company, Vickers/Medelec Limited. About 2 in 3 North American ECT clinics are equipped with Mecta machines.

The reliability of the British sales and maintenance service is unknown, but Medelec/Vickers do have a good national reputation.

MECTA SR1, SR2, JR1 AND JR2 MODELS

Year of manufacture   1985 to current. 'British' models introduced 1993
Price at June 1994   SR1 and SR2: £7770 (excl. VAT)
JR1 and JR2: £3932 (excl. VAT)
Dimensions   SR models: 17 cm × 47 cm × 35 cm; 17.7 kg; metal casing
JR models: 17 cm × 13 cm × 35 cm; 9.6 kg; metal casing

Description

SR models differ from JR models in that they have built-in dual channel monitoring. Machines are manufactured on a modular basis, so the monitoring modules can be interchanged to give any combination of ECG or EEG monitoring (e.g. single channel ECG and EEG, or dual channel EEG). JR models can be upgraded to the corresponding SR model by addition of monitoring and recording modules which fit together inside the SR chassis. The practical difference between 1 and 2 model designations is that SR2/JR2 models have a single output control dial – where stimulus parameters are predetermined by the manufacturer – while SR1/JR1 models offer independent control over four brief-pulse stimulus parameters (current, pulse width, frequency and stimulus duration).

Machines are controlled by a microprocessor, so they can be customised or upgraded without having to purchase a new machine. Only the microprocessor is replaced.

'British' and 'International' (IEC) Mectas (see below) are essentially customised versions of the corresponding 'US domestic versions' (i.e. machines in use in the US).

An important technical difference between 'US domestic' SR1/JR1 and SR2/JR2 models is that stimulus intensity (in mC/s) is generally lower in Series 2 models, and stimulus duration is extremely short at the lower end of the output range. 'US domestic' SR2/JR2 models are not suited to seizure threshold titration. The manufacturers have improved the predetermined stimulus parameter values of British SR2/JR2 models at low output settings, and these values now correspond closely to the settings for SR1/JR1 models when following the seizure threshold stimulation schedule which is widely used in North America (see Chapter 22). 'British' Mecta SR2/JR2 models are now well suited to seizure threshold titration. 'British' Mectas also have an increased maximum power output (1200 mC) compared with their American (576 mC max) and IEC (403 mC max) counterparts.

SR1

SR2

(1)   Mains on/off switch with indicator light
(2)   Stimulus control dial
    (a) for pulse width
    (b) for frequency
    (c) for stimulus duration
    (d) for current strength
(3)   Self-test on/off button with indicator light
(4)   Treat on/off button with indicator light
(5)   SR2/JR2 'British' – high range switch; US Domestic – impedance override switch
(6)   Electrode connector sockets
(7a)   LCD display of dose delivered
(7b)   Display panel intensity dial
(8)   Socket for EEG monitor lead
(9)   Interchangeable ECG or EEG modules
(10)   On/off switch for dual channel chart recorder
(11)   On/off switches for respective channel monitors
(12)   Dual channel chart recorder
(13)-(19)
    Dials and switches specific to monitoring and/or operation of the chart recorder

Stimulus characteristics

Waveform: Biphasic brief-pulse.
Stimulus characteristics: These are given separately for the different versions. All machines work on the constant current principle at given predetermined current settings throughout the output range up to 400 Ω load. Voltage varies with impedance; maximum voltage 240 V.

British version JR2/SR2
    Pulse width = automatically varied from 1.0–1.4 ms
    Frequency = automatically varied from 40–90 Hz
    Current = automatically varied from 550–800 mA
    Stimulus duration = automatically varied from 0.55–6.00 s
    Output range: 25–1200 mC, divided into low range (25–400 mC; 25 mC increments) and high range (450–1200 mC; 50 mC increments); maximum stimulus intensity 202 mC/s.

British version JR1/SR1
    Pulse width (6 switch settings) = 1.0, 1.2, 1.4, 1.6, 1.8, 2.0 ms
    Frequency (6 switch settings) = 40, 50, 60, 70, 80, 90 Hz
    Current (6 switch settings) = 550, 600, 650, 700, 750, 800 mA
    Stimulus duration (10 settings) = 0.5, 0.75, 1.0, 1.25, 1.5, 2.0, 2.5, 3.0, 3.5, 4.0 s
    Output range: 22 mC to 1152 mC; maximum stimulus intensity 288 mC/s

International (IEC) version JR2/SR2
    Pulse width = fixed at 1.0 ms
    Frequency = fixed at 90 Hz
    Current = fixed at 800 mA
    Stimulus duration = automatically varied from 0.16–2.85.
    Output range = 22.4–403.2 mC (2.5–71.0 at 220 Ω; 3.5–96.8 J at 300 Ω)
    Maximum stimulus intensity 144 mC/s.

International (IEC) version JR1/SR1
    Pulse width (5 switch settings) = 1.0, 1.1, 1.2, 1.3, 1.4 ms.
    Frequency (6 switch settings) = 40, 50, 60, 70, 80, 90 Hz
    Current (6 switch settings) = 550, 600, 650, 700, 750, 800 mA.
    Stimulus duration (6 switch settings) - 0.5, 0.75, 1.0, 2.25, 2.05 ms.
    Ouput range = 22.0–403 mC (2.7–71.0 J at 220 Ω; 3.6–98.8 J at 300 Ω).
    Maximum stimulus intensity 202 mC/s.

US domestic version JR2/SR2
    Pulse width (fixed) = 1.0 ms
    Frequency (fixed) = 90 Hz
    Current (fixed) = 800 mA
    Stimulus duration (256 equal space steps) = 0.1–4.0 s
    Output range = 22 mC to 576 mC; maximum stimulus intensity 144 mC.

US domestic version JR1/SR1
    Pulse width (6 switch settings) = 1.0, 1.2, 1.4, 1.6, 1.8, 2.0 ms
    Frequency (6 switch settings) = 40, 50, 60, 70, 80, 90 Hz
    Current (6 switch settings) = 550, 600, 650, 700, 750, 800 mA
    Stimulus duration (6 switch settings) = 0.5, 0.75, 1.0, 1.25, 1.5, 2.0 s
    Output range: 22–576 mC; maximum stimulus intensity 288 mC/s.

Output display (all versions)

Outcome of self-test, notification of functional status, set dose and dose actually delivered are given sequentially on the LCD display screen. SR models automatically print the dose actually delivered, dynamic impedance and stimulus parameter values.

Safety features (all versions)

The machines have a 'self-test' function for measuring static impedance, and an automatic stimulus abort function. A warning (both audible and visual) is given prior to the passage of stimulus, and the treatment stimulus is accompanied by a continuous tone and a message on the LCD display screen. Stimulation is automatically prevented under conditions of high impedance. It is possible to proceed with the stimulation by using the 'impedance override' button on US domestic versions, but this override function is not available on British versions. Machines are constructed to American (CSA), German (TUV) and International (IEC 601-1) safety standards.[11]

Input supply

SR and JRI models must be connected to a transformer which is then connected to the British mains supply. JR2i models connect directly to the British mains supply.

Other

A comprehensive manual and instructive videotapes are provided by the manufacturer. The manufacturers have produced customised hand-held electrodes with an optional remote control treat button. With Mecta electrodes, electrode-to-patient contact is achieved by means of electrolyte paste or gel, rather than by the traditional method of moistening the electrode with fluid, which should not be used.

Comments

Information provided by the manufacturer
Dose titration guidelines are provided for JRI and SRI models.

The North American videos supplied by the manufacturer are to be avoided, as they contain references to ECT administration and monitoring techniques of no scientific or practical merit.

Other
Mecta (and Thymatron – see below) machines incorporate many features which are not available on comparable British machines, and it is not necessary for a trained third party to trigger the stimulus from the machine itself. Compared with the Thymatron the main practical advantages of 'British' SR2/JR2 models include the ease of access to the high dose range, and the manner in which the control dial is calibrated. The main disadvantage of the Mecta SR2 is that it is cumbersome, and the daunting array of buttons and dials on the monitoring and chart recording modules detracts from the simplicity of use of the ECT stimulation module. The advantage of the modular system of construction is that a JR unit can be upgraded at a later stage to the corresponding SR unit. Like Thymatron, but unlike all British machines, upgrading Mecta machines does not necessitate the purchase of a new machine. All that is required is a new microprocessor, which can be fitted 'on-site'.

---

11. The adminidstration of a stimulus dose in excess of 504 mC is inconsistent with IEC 606-1.

SR2 models are suited to clinics wanting to adopt EEG monitoring; JR2 models are otherwise recommended. SR1/JR1 models are suited to clinics with a specific research interest in brief-pulse stimulation characteristics. Customised 'British' versions are preferable to international (IEC) and US domestic versions, as the maximum output of the latter may be insufficient for patients with high seizure thresholds, and the predetermined stimulus parameters of IEC and US JR2 /SR2 models do not facilitate accurate threshold titration in patients with low seizure thresholds.

Reliable threshold titration guidelines are available for JR1 and SR1 models (see Chapter 22). Two members of the ECT Committee (Dr Toni Lock and Dr Alan Scott) are presently using British version SR2 machines. Guidelines for stimulus dosing using British version JR2/SR2 machines are given on page 83, based on experience in the Broadoak Psychiatric Unit and Mossley Hill Hospital.

Rankings ('British' models): (1 = best; 7 = worst)

Safety:	1
Stimulus parameters:	1
Output range:	1
Ease of use:	1 (SR2/JR2) or 6 (SR1/JR1)
Dose titration:	1
After sales:	too early to tell
Price:	5 (SR2) 4 (JR2)

Machines manufactured by Somatics Incorporated, US

Address	910 Sherwood Drive, Unit 17, Lake Bluff, Illinois 60044, US
	Telephone (US) 313 2346761
Sales and maintenance	Dantec, Techno House, Redcliffe Way, Bristol BS1 6NU
	Telephone 01179 291436
	Fax 01179 213532

Thymatron machines were developed in 1985 by two American psychiatrists, Abrams and Swartz, in collaboration with electronic engineers. The original Thymatron machine was upgraded to the present Thymatron-DG model in 1989. About 1 in 3 North American ECT clinics are equipped with Thymatron machines. Somatics Incorporated began to market their products in Britain in 1992 through the British medical instrument company, Dantec Limited. The reliability of the British sales and maintenance service is unknown, but Dantec has a good national reputation.

THYMATRON-DGx

Year of manufacture	1989 to current. 'British' modified flexi-dial introduced in 1993
Price at June 1994	£7950 (excl. VAT) for complete unit with EEG printer; £5150 (excl. VAT) for unit without EEG printer
Dimensions	For complete unit, 10.9 × 38.5 × 28.6 cm; weight 10 kg; metal casing (unit without EEG printer, 10.9 × 24 × 28.6 cm; weight 7.2 kg)

Description

The machine comprises an ECT stimulus unit and a printer unit which fit together. The stimulus unit can be purchased separately. The machine is controlled by a microprocessor which means that it can be upgraded without having to purchase a new machine: only the microprocessor is replaced.

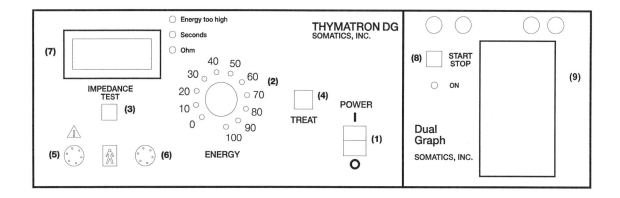

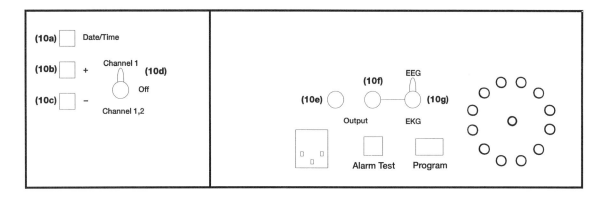

(1)   Mains on/off switch with indicator light
(2)   Stimulus control dial
(3)   Impedance test button
(4)   Treat button
(5)   Electrode connector socket
(6)   Patient monitor connector socket
(7)   Digital display panel for dose delivered and impedance
(8)   On/off switch for chart recorder
(9)   Chart recorder
(10) Dials and switches specific to monitoring and/or operation of the chart recorder

The Thymatron has a single stimulus output control dial, calibrated in percentages of maximum output, which automatically varies several stimulus parameters. A special accessory, the 'Flexi-Dial stimulus controller', plugs into the back of the machine and allows the operator to override predetermined pulse frequency and pulse width parameters. The Flexi-Dial has been adapted for British use by the addition of an 'Energy × 2' setting. When operating in normal mode (i.e. without Flexi-Dial attachment or with Flexi-Dial attached but switched to the 'preset' setting), British Thymatrons are identical to the machines used in North American clinics, with a maximum output of 504 mC. When the Flexi-Dial is set to the Energy × 2 setting, the output at each percentage setting on the control dial is doubled. For example, at the 50% setting, 252 mC (50% × 504 mC) will be delivered when the machine is operating in normal mode, and 504 mC (50% × 1007 mC) in 'Flexi-Dial Energy × 2' mode. An 'Alarm' switch on the Flexi-Dial must be turned off before the machine will deliver a stimulus in excess of 504 mC.

Stimulus characteristics

Waveform: Biphasic brief-pulse.
Pulse width: Fixed (i.e. non-variable) at 1.0 ms in normal mode. Fixed at 1.5 ms in 'Flexi-Dial Energy × 2' mode. Flexi-Dial options: 0.5, 1.0 and 1.5 ms.

Current: Constant at 900 mA throughout the output range, up to a 500 Ω impedance load. Voltage varies with dynamic impedance; maximum voltage 450 V. Current cannot be varied by means of the 'Flexi-Dial' accessory.
Pulse frequency: Automatically varied from 30 to 70 Hz in 'normal' mode; fixed at 70 Hz in 'Flexi-Dial Energy × 2' mode.
Flexi-Dial options: 30, 40, 50, 60, 70 Hz.
Stimulus duration: Automatically varied from 0.47 to 4 seconds in 'normal' mode; and from 0.26 to 5.3 seconds in 'Flexi-Dial Energy × 2' mode.
Output range: 25–504 mC (normal range); 504–1007 mC ('Flexi-Dial Energy × 2' range).

Output control

A single dial is calibrated in percentages (5–100%, in units of 5%). Each 5% energy increase is approximately equal to 25.2 mC (normal range) or 50.4 mC ('Flexi-Dial Energy × 2' range).

Output display

The dose actually delivered is displayed on a digital display panel. Time (in seconds) is displayed on the digital display screen from when the treatment button is released, thus offering the operator a reliable means of measuring seizure duration without having to use a timing device. Several computer/automated measures are automatically printed at the end of each ECT treatment: EEG and/or EMG end point, 'seizure energy index', 'post-ictal suppression index', and 'seizure concordance index'.

Monitoring

The machine incorporates audible EEG monitoring, as the machine converts the EEG signal to an auditory signal. The dual channel printer can be set (on the back of the machine) to give any combination of ECG, EEG or EMG (electromyograph). An additional fee must be paid for the EMG option.

Safety features

The machine has an impedance test function, and indicates the passage of current both audibly and visually. It provides a warning that the stimulus is about to be passed, and has two automatic stimulus abort functions. The first is under control of the treat button, which may be prematurely released to abort the stimulus; the second is a unique safety circuit independent of the regular circuit, which prevents the administration of a stimulus which varies by more than 5% from the selected value. When triggered, the alarm circuit emits a wavering alarm tone and the stimulus is automatically aborted. The treatment button is protected by a hard plastic cover which prevents it from being accidentally depressed. The machine is certified to CSA, TUV and IEC 601-1 standards.[12]

Instruction manuals, a videotape and an audio cassette are supplied with each machine. The manufacturer has produced customised hand-held electrodes, which are suited to the 'traditional' method of establishing patient-to-electrode contact.

Input supply

Machines can be connected directly to the British mains (240 V, 60 Hz, AC) or North American mains (110 V, 40 Hz, AC) supply.

12. An output of greater than 504 mC is incompatible with IEC 606-1.

Comments

Information supplied by the manufacturer

The 'post-ictal suppression index' concept has been patented. The computer automated measures of seizure adequacy are based on physiological markers which are associated with therapeutic seizures, but their reliability and validity has been questioned. These measures have still to be fully evaluated and should not be used as an alternative to sound clinical judgement.

The guidelines for stimulus dosing in the instruction manual are to select the percentage dial setting which most closely corresponds to the age of a patient. This dosing strategy is simplistic, and not appropriate for bilateral ECT. The dose titration strategy devised for Mecta SR1 machines has been adapted for users of Thymatron machines (see Chapter 22).

Other

Thymatron (and Mecta – see above) machines incorporate many features which are not included on British machines, and it is not necessary for a trained third party to trigger the stimulus from the machine itself. The audible EEG function of the Thymatron has limited practical value.

The main practical differences between Mecta JR1/JR2 and Thymatron models relate to the ease of access to the high dose range, and the manner in which the control dial is calibrated. With the Thymatron, the 'Flexi-Dial' accessory must be plugged in and set to the 'Energy × 2' setting, and the alarm circuit must be switched off before the machine will deliver a stimulus in excess of 504 mC. Having to undertake the latter procedure when a patient is anaesthetised and has already had one or more stimulations at the maximum output setting in 'normal' mode is extremely impractical. The alternative is to use the machine permanently connected to the 'Flexi-Dial; which would be switched to the 'Preset' setting for outputs up to 504 mC, and the 'Energy × 2' setting for ouputs in excess of 504 mC. The operator must remember whether the machine is operating in normal or extended dose ranges and must remember to activate or de-activate the alarm switch on the Flexi-Dial. This increases the risk of operator error with respect to selecting an appropriate stimulus dose.

Predetermined stimulus parameters of Thymatron models were superior to those of US domestic Mecta SR2 and JR2 models, and Thymatron machines performed better at the low output settings necessary for seizure threshold titration strategies. This is no longer the case with British Mecta SR2/JR2 models. The technical disadvantage of the 'Energy × 2' modification of the US domestic machine is that there is not a smooth transition of predetermined stimulus parameter values between 'normal' (25.2–504 mC) and extended (504–1007 mC) output ranges.

Like Mecta, but unlike British machines, upgrading Thymatron machines does not necessitate the purchase of a new machine. All that is required is a new microprocessor, which can be fitted 'on site'.

Reliable dose titration guidelines (see page 86) are available. Two members of the ECT Committee (Susan Benbow and Toni Lock) are presently using these machines.

Rankings: (1 = best; 7 = worst)

Safety:	1
Stimulus parameters:	1
Output range:	1
Ease of use:	2 (without flexi-dial), 4 (with flexi-dial)
Dose titration:	1
After-sales:	Too early to tell
Price:	6

Selection criteria

Local factors

Local factors to consider when selecting a new machine include:

(1) the standard of expertise of ECT clinic staff;
(2) the time available to the Consultant in charge of ECT for the training and supervision of the staff who actually administer the treatment;
(3) the nature of on-going or proposed research and audit projects, if any;
(4) the age range of patients treated in the clinic;
(5) the number of patients;
(6) budgetary constraints.

Safety considerations

Test for static impedance

The major determinants of static impedance are: (1) the contact achieved between ECT electrodes and the scalp; and (2) the cranium and covering tissues. Poor electrode-to-patient contact may result in an excessively high output voltage to maintain current at a constant level, which may predispose to electrical arcing and skin burns – particularly when the patient's head becomes wet from excessive electrode solution dribbling from pre-soaked electrodes. At high impedance values, the machine may not be able to maintain current at a constant level and the patient may be at risk of receiving a stimulus which fails to induce an adequate seizure. It is therefore important to ensure that static impedance values are within the acceptable range for the given machine before proceeding to stimulate the patient. (Dynamic impedance can only be measured once current is passing through the brain, but is only a fraction of static impedance.) All shortlisted models incorporate a test function for measuring static impedance: the 'Test' function on Ectron Series 5A machines; the 'Self-Test' on Mecta models; and the 'Impedance test' on the Thymatron.

Automatic stimulus abort function

It may occasionally be necessary to abort the passage of current in the event of an emergency. With American-made machines, this is possible by premature release of the 'treat' button. Stimulus duration is otherwise automatically terminated when pressure on the treat button is maintained. With British-made machines, the only ways in which the passage of current may be aborted once the 'treat' button has been depressed is to remove the electrodes from the patient's head (which may result in electrical arcing and skin burns), or if a trained third party is standing by, to switch off the machine promptly. It is therefore recommended that a trained third party triggers the stimulus from the machine itself.

Indication of patient stimulation

It is important to be warned beforehand that the electrical stimulus is about to be passed, and to the actual passage of the stimulus. American machines do both, while British machines only alert the operator to the actual passage of the stimulus. Indication of patient stimulation should be audible and visible.

Independent laboratory certification

Machines should be constructed with regard to British Safety Standard BS 5724 'General Requirements for Electromedical Equipment'. Parts 1 and 2 of BS 5724 deal specifically with ECT machines. The absence of BS 5724 certification does not imply that the machine is unsafe, or that it its use is illegal in Britain. CSA (USA and Canada), TUV (German), and International (IEC 601) safety approval is compatible with British safety standards, and machines with TUV certification may be used throughout the EEC.

Stimulus parameters

The machine should generate a brief-pulse waveform and should operate on the constant current principle within a specified range of impedance values. It is generally accepted that biphasic brief-pulse stimulation is preferable to uniphasic stimulation. The maximum voltage response to high impedance values should be limited for safety reasons. The most valid measure of stimulus output (or 'dose') is in units of electrical charge, millicoulombs (mC). As the same amount of charge (in mC) may be delivered over different periods of time, the rate at which charge is delivered (mC/s) indicates the stimulus intensity.

There is no scientific evidence to suggest that sine-wave stimulation is likely to succeed when brief-pulse stimulation has failed to induce seizures and/or effect symptomatic relief.

Pulse width, pulse frequency, current and stimulus duration values should be within the upper and lower limits quoted in Table 4 throughout the entire output range. These criteria have not been met by any manufacturer, but certain deficits are more important than others. Optimum values at given output settings remain to be determined, and it remains uncertain as to whether or not there exists a dominant parameter. Predetermined values (in the case of single control machines) differ from one model to the next at equivalent output settings. It is therefore invalid to compare dosages (in mC) in absolute terms. The stimulus parameter options on multiple control machines also differ from one model to the next. This makes it difficult to adapt stimulus dosing strategies developed for one multiple control machine for use with another.

Output

Output range

The International (IEC 601-1) standard limits the output of an ECT machine to about 500 mC, the reasons for which are unclear and the subject of international debate. Administering an output dose in excess of this figure voids IEC and TUV safety approval. We, nevertheless, recommend that ECT machines should be capable of putting out a charge of at least 1000 mC, as we are of the opinion that stimulating patients in the 500–1200 mC range is justified in approximately 5% to 10% of cases, when patients fail to have adequate seizures at output levels under 500 mC despite hyperventilation with oxygen (see Chapter 15). The alternative to increasing the stimulus dose is augmentation with neuronal stimulants (e.g. intravenous caffeine and/or theophylline), which is also not without risk. The comparative safety of 'high' output doses versus pharmacological augmentation techniques remains to be determined.

For the purposes of dose titration of low seizure threshold patients, a minimum output of no greater than 25 mC is recommended in a time of no less than 0.5 seconds. (Seizures are not reliably induced if stimulus duration is less than 0.5 seconds.) Small dose increments of approximately 25 mC are necessary. Larger dose increments (e.g. 50 mC) are acceptable at the high end of the output range. Another factor to consider is stimulus intensity, which should increase at a uniform rate from minimum to maximum output settings.

Output control

ECT machines must offer the operator a means of varying the stimulus output. As the dose of a brief-pulse stimulus is determined by phase, pulse width, pulse frequency, stimulus duration, and current strength, stimulus output may be controlled by one or more of these parameters. Stimulus parameters at different output settings are predetermined by the manufacturer and are automatically varied in the case of single control dial machines.

Multiple control machines offer independent control over two or more brief-pulse stimulus parameters. The Thymatron can be converted from a single control to a multiple control machine by means of a special accessory.

Output display

The machine should display the dose which was actually delivered to the patient, as this may differ from the dose which the machine was set to deliver under conditions of high static and/or dynamic impedance. A difference of more than 5% is significant, and suggests poor technique and/or faulty equipment. Machines with built-in monitoring automatically print the dose delivered, stimulus parameter settings at that dose, and dynamic impedance values.

Ease of use

Single control machines are considerably more 'user-friendly' than multiple control machines, and are recommended for routine NHS clinical work. Multiple control machines demand a greater degree of technical expertise, training and supervision if they are to be used competently and present a higher risk of clinical error in inexperienced hands. Multiple control machines are best reserved for clinics with a specific research interest in brief-pulse stimulus parameter characteristics. Single control machines would be adequate for all other research and audit projects.

Single control machines which are calibrated in millicoulombs (e.g. Ectron Series 5A, Mecta SR2/JR2 models) are the easiest to operate and present the least risk of dosing errors.

It is time consuming to have to convert percentage output of total into millicoulombs for record keeping purposes (e.g. Thymatron) and even more tedious to have to calculate output (e.g. Neurotronic machines).

EEG monitoring also demands a higher investment of training and supervision time if the facility is to be used competently, but offers valuable training experience relevant to seizure disorders in general. Monitoring is considered advantageous, but not essential, so has been excluded from the 'ease of use' ratings.

Whether or not a machine connects directly to the British mains supply (240 V, 60 Hz, AC) or to a transformer (which converts the British mains supply to 110 V, 40 Hz, AC) is irrelevant with respect to safety or ease of use. The only disadvantage of a transformer is that it takes up space.

Dose titration

Considerable information on seizure threshold titration and stimulus dosing strategies is available for Mecta SR1 and JR1 models, based on North American experience. These policies have been adapted for use with the Thymatron and 'British' Mecta SR2 and JR2 models. Relatively limited information is available for Ectron Series 5A and Neurotronic machines, and what information is available is based on anecdotal experience. Dosing policies have been developed for these machines and are given in Chapter 22.

After sales service

Reliable service from the manufacturer or agent is important with respect to repairs and maintenance. The after-sales service provided by Ectron Limited is known to be reliable, while that for the other shortlisted machines remains to be put to the test. Ectron Limited have traditionally demanded that ECT machines be returned to them for servicing. A 'maintenance contract', which guarantees on-site service within a specified period of time can be arranged for the Mecta and Thymatron machines. The cost of such a maintenance contract is significant, but should be offset against the need for two new machines – if the main (new) machine could be guaranteed to be back in action for the next ECT clinic day, then an existing (old) machine would be adequate as a back-up.

Price

An ECT machine is probably the only item of 'high-tech' medical equipment which is requested by psychiatrists, and the price of an ECT machine should be regarded as the least important selection criteria. A maintenance contract could cut the cost of re-equipping an ECT clinic by 50% (reasons above). Built-in EEG monitoring more than doubles the cost of an ECT machine, and there is a recurring cost of consumables (recording paper and disposable electrodes) of approximately £4.00 per patient for a course of treatment.

Because American models are based on a microprocessor, they offer the advantage of being able to be upgraded at a later stage without having to purchase a new machine. The write-down cost of most electrical medical equipment is three years: ECT machines should be no different.

Electrodes

In North America, ECT electrodes are flat metal plates which are strapped to a patient's head by a rubber band. British psychiatrists have traditionally used hand-held electrodes, and there is no good reason to change to the American method. Hand-held electrodes suitable to British practice should be sturdy and well insulated, and should offer a firm grip. The operator's hand should be protected from inadvertently making contact with the live end of the electrodes. Calliper-type electrodes are obsolete. A long retractable cable enables the machine to be positioned anywhere in the room. All ranked models now come equipped with suitable electrodes, as both American manufacturers have produced customised hand-held electrodes for the British market.

In North America, electrode-to-patient contact is achieved by means of electrolyte paste or gel, while the 'traditional' British method is to soak the (padded) ends of the electrodes in an electrolyte solution. Either method is acceptable. There is some evidence to suggest that static impedance values are lower with the paste/gel method, and that there is a lower incidence of skin burns.

Patient monitoring

Built-in ECG monitoring offers little practical advantage, as most British ECT clinics are equipped with portable ECG machines, or combined ECG/cardiac defibrillators. Dual channel EEG monitoring is of direct patient benefit in a small minority of cases, for example, where, due to high levels of muscle relaxant, it is not clear whether a fit has occurred or where prolonged cerebral seizure activity is suspected.

The problem is that such cases cannot be predicted beforehand so, if EEG monitoring is to be of benefit to a small minority of patients when the need arises, it needs to be undertaken on all or the majority of clinic patients. Single channel EEG recording is subject to artefact and is not recommended.

The recurring cost of EEG monitoring can be reduced by using cheap disposable paediatric ECG electrodes, which are suitable for EEG monitoring.

References

PIPPARD, J. (1992) Audit of electroconvulsive treatment in two National Health Service regions. *British Journal of Psychiatry*, **160**, 621–637.
ROYAL COLLEGE OF PSYCHIATRISTS (1994) *Electroconvulsive Therapy (ECT). The Official Video Teaching Pack of the Royal College of Psychiatrists' Special Committee on ECT*. London: Royal College of Psychiatrists.
RUSSELL, R. J. (1988) Stimuli used in ECT. In *Current Approaches: ECT* (eds J. C. Malkin & S. Brandon), pp. 58–60. Southampton: Duphar Medical Relations.
STEPHENS, S. M., GREENBERG, R. M. & PETTINATI, H. M. (1991) Choosing an electroconvulsive therapy device. *Psychiatric Clinics of North America: Electroconvulsive Therapy*, **14**, 989–1006.

Index
Compiled by Caroline Sheard

adolescent patients 18–21
adverse effects
    cognitive 68–69
    medical 67–68
    psychiatric 68
    psychological 69
    recommendations 70
alcohol 55
Alzheimer's disease 26
amantadine 12
amenorrhoea 67
amitriptyline 50, 51
amnesia 68–69
amoxapine 50
anaemia 44
anaesthesia 42
    contraindications 43–44
    equipment 46–47
    induction agents 45
    investigations preceding 42–43
    muscle relaxants 45–46
    patient assessment 42
    premedication 44
    preparation for 44
    recovery from 47
    repeated 31
    ventilation during 46
aneurysm
    aortic 27, 43
    intracranial 27
anorexia 67
anterograde amnesia 68
anticholinergics 12
anticoagulant therapy 27
anticonvulsants 44, 53–54
antidepressant drug therapy 49–50
    in combination with ECT 44, 49–50
    comparison with ECT 3
    continuation after ECT 4, 58
antipsychotic drugs, comparison with
    ECT 6
antisocial behaviour 9, 30
aortic aneurysm 27, 43
ASA rating 27
aspiration pneumonia 67
atropine 44
aversive shock treatment 32

battery 97
BECT 60–61, 72–73
benzodiazepines 12, 44, 49
beta-adrenoceptor antagonists (b–blockers)
    44, 52–53
bilateral ECT 60–61, 72–73
bite block 45
bladder rupture 68
brain damage 4, 69
breast-feeding 23
brief-pulse stimulation 68, 72, 88, 89
    calculating charge for 90
bromocriptine 12

caffeine 26, 44, 54–55
capnograph 47
carbamazepine 54
cardiac arrhythmias 13
cardiac pacemakers 27, 43
cardiovascular disease 27
    and anaesthesia 43
catatonia 11
    acute states 9
cerebral tumours 43
cervical spine disease 28
charge 88–89, 90
children as patients 19
chlorpromazine 8, 9, 53
chopped sine-waveform 88, 89
chronic subdural haematoma 27
clomipramine 51
clonic phase 62
clovoxamine 50
clozapine 53
compulsory ECT 99
confusional states 15, 68, 69
consent 97–98
    adolescents 19
    by relatives 99
    and emergency ECT 98–99
    form 113
    patient incapable of giving or with-
        holding 98
    refusal 98
    Republic of Ireland 99–100
    and sham ECT 31
constant current 91, 92

constant energy 91
constant voltage 91
continuation ECT 71
Cotard's syndrome 24
craniotomy, ECT following 27
Creuzfeldt–Jakob disease 26
Criminal Procedure (Scotland) Act 1975 97
cuff technique 63, 64

dantrolene 12
delirium, post-ictal 69
delusions
    depressive 3
    persecutory 9
dementing illnesses 26
dentures 45
depressive disorders 3–5
    in childhood and adolescence 18
    in mental handicap 24
    post-stroke 26
desmethylimipramine 50
detained patients and consent 98, 99
diabetes mellitus 33, 44
diazepam 45, 49
discontinuation of treatment 3–4
dopaminomimetic psychosis 9
dose 88–89, 90
    moderately suprathreshold 74–75
    predetermined 77
    standard 72
    strategy at first treatment session 77–78
    therapeutic window 74–75
    titration 31–32, 77–83, 147
    see also stimulus dosing
Down's syndrome 24, 27
doxepin 50
droperidol 53
drowsiness 67
drugs 40–41, 47, 49–57
dynamic impedance 91–92

E-delta-2-VAP 54
ECG monitoring 27, 47, 148
ECT suite 37
    equipment 39–41
    recent trends 37–38
    shared facilities 37–38
    staffing 38
Ectron Mark 4 72, 131–132
    features 123, 124
Ectron Series 2 72, 129–130
    features 123, 124
Ectron Series 3 72, 129–130
    features 123, 124
Ectron Series 5 128–129

features 123, 124
    waveform 90
Ectron Series 5A 32, 122, 126–128
    dose titration protocol 78–80
    features 123, 124
    stimulus dosing schedule 83
    waveform 90
EEG monitoring 62, 64–66, 148
Elcot machines 122
elderly patients 17
    anaesthesia 43
electric shock treatment, non-convulsive 31–32
electrodes 148
    d'Elia position 72
    Lancaster position 72
    placement 60–61
emergencies
    and consent 98–99
    drugs for 40–41, 47
    equipment for 40
epilepsy 15–16, 26–27
equipment 39–41
    anaesthetic 46–47
    maintenance 40
    review of machines 122–148
ethanol 55
etomidate 45
extrapyramidal syndromes, drug-induced 14–15

factsheet 103–105
    out-patients 106
fake ECT 31
families
    and consent 99
    factsheet 103–105
fluoxetine 50, 51
fluphenazine 53
fluvoxamine 50–51
foetus, effects of maternal ECT 22–23
frequency of treatment 58
    in depressive disorders 4
    in mania 6
Friedreich's ataxia 27
fugue states 15

gastroparesis 67–68
glaucoma 43
glycopyrrolate 44

hallucinations, depressive 3
haloperidol 53
headache 67
Huntington's chorea 26

hyperkalaemia 13
hypertension 43
hypoglycaemic drugs 44
hypoxaemia 46

ibuprofen 67
imipramine 3, 50, 51
insulin coma 8
intellectual impairment following ECT 4

joules 88

L-dopa 12
L-tryptophan 53
lactation 23
lamotrigine 54
latent phase 62
LC 11, 12, 13
learning disability 24–25, 27
legal aspects 97–100
lethal catatonia 11, 12, 13
lignocaine 45
literature bias 13
lithium 52
    comparison with ECT 6

machines
    after sales service 147–148
    automatic stimulus abort function 145
    dose titration 147
    ease of use 147
    independent laboratory certification 145
    indication of patient stimulation 145
    models 122–144
    monitoring facilities 148
    output control and display 146–147
    price 148
    safety considerations 145–146
    selection criteria 145–148
    self test function 76
    stimulus parameters 146
    test for static impedance 145
maintenance ECT 71
malignant hyperthermia 11, 12, 43
mania 6–7, 68
    in childhood and adolescence 18
maprotiline 50
Mecta JR1 137–141
    features 123, 124, 125
    stimulus dosing schedule 83
Mecta JR2 137–141
    features 123, 124, 125
    stimulus dosing schedule 83
Mecta SR1 137–141
    features 123, 124, 125

    stimulus dosing schedule 83, 86–87
Mecta SR2 137–141
    features 123, 124, 125
    stimulus dosing schedule 83
medazolam 49, 69
Medcraft machines 122
memory impairment 68–69
Mental Health Act 1983 19, 97
Mental Health (Northern Ireland) Order 1946 19, 97
Mental Health (Scotland) Act 1984 19, 97
Mental Treatment Act 1945 (Republic of Ireland) 99
methohexitone 45
metoclopramide 53
MH 11, 12, 43
mianserin 50, 51
mivacurium 46
moclobemide 51
monitoring 62–66
    equipment 39, 46–47
monoamine oxidase inhibitors 44, 50, 51–52
mortality 67
muscle aches 67
muscle relaxants 45–46
muscular dystrophy 43
myasthenia gravis 43
myocardial infarction 27, 43
myocardial ischaemia 43
myopathy 43

nausea 67
neuroleptic drugs 8–9, 53
    extrapyramidal side-effects 14–15
neuroleptic malignant sydrome 9, 11, 12–14
neurosyphilis 27
Neurotronic Therapy System machines 132–136
    dose titration protocols 80–82
    features 123, 124
nicotine 55
NMS 9, 11, 12–14
non-convulsive electric shock treatment 31–32
normal pressure hydrocephalus 26
nursing guidelines 114–121

obesity 44
obsessive–compulsive disorder 33–34
obstetrics 22–23
OCD 33–34
oesophageal reflux 44
offending behaviour 9, 30

Ohm's Law 88
One Flew over the Cuckoo's Nest 32
out-patients, factsheet 106

Paget's disease of the skull 27
paranoid syndromes 9
Parkinson's disease 12
paroxetine 51
patients
    elderly 17, 43
    factsheets 103–106
    pre-anaesthetic assessment 42
    preparation 44
    young 18–21
phaeochromocytoma 43
phencyclidine psychosis 9
phenelzine 3
phenobarbitone 54
phenothiazines 8
physical illness 26–29
placebo ECT 31
polyspike activity 62, 66
post-ictal confusional states 15
postpartum psychosis 23
predictors of good response 3
pregnancy 22–23, 44
premedication 44
prescribing 3, 58–59
procyclidine 14
promethazine 53
prophylactic ECT 71
propofol 45
propranolol 52
psychomotor retardation 3
pulse oximeter 47

raised intracranial pressure 27, 43
record form 107–112
recovery room 37, 47
    equipment 39
relapse
    depressive disorders 4
    rate of 58
Republic of Ireland, consent 99–100
retrograde amnesia 68

schizoaffective disorders 9
schizophrenia 8
    in childhood and adolescence 18
    drug-resistant 8
    recommendations 9
    type I 8–9
    type II 8
    and violence 30

schizophreniform disorders, drug-induced 9
seizure
    duration 76
    missed/failed 62, 65, 74, 93
    neurophysiology of induction 92–93
    partial 62, 74, 93
    prolonged 64, 67
    qualitative differences in 93
    spontaneous 67
    tardive 67
    timing 62–63, 64
seizure threshold 73–74
    in adolescents 20
    change over course of treatment 63, 73
    in elderly 17
    factors affecting 74
    units 73
selective serotonin reuptake inhibitors 50–51
sertraline 51
sham ECT 31
sickle-cell disease 44
sickle-cell trait 44
Siemens Konvulsator 122
sine-wave stimulation 68, 72, 88, 89
SLE NTS-C 135–136
SLE NTS-R 133–135
sodium valproate 54
spike-and-wave activity 62, 66
spine, cervical, unstable disease 28
SSRIs 50–51
staff
    medical 38
    nursing 38
    training and supervision 46, 94
staffing 38
static impedance 91–92, 145
status epilepticus 15
steroids 12
stimulus dosing 31–32, 72–73, 147
    examples 78–83, 86–87
    guidelines for developing a policy 76–78
    policy 84–86
stimulus intensity 89, 91
stimulus waveform 88, 89, 90
stroke 26, 43
subconvulsive stimulations 31–32
succinylcholine 13
sulpiride 53
supervision 94
suxamethonium 45–46

TCAs 44, 49–50
teeth, loose 68
therapeutic window 74–75

thiopentone 45
thioridazine 13, 53
thrombophlebitis 43
Thymatron-DGX 141–144
   features 123, 125
   predetermined dose at first treatment session 77
   stimulus dosing schedule 83, 86–87
timing, seizures 62–63, 64
tonic phase 62
toxic delirium 52
training 94
treatment record form 107–112
treatment room 37
triangular waveform 88, 89
tricyclic antidepressants 44, 49–50
trifluperidol 53
triple-pulse waveform 90
trisomy 21 24, 27

twilight states 15

UECT 60–61, 72
ultra-brief-pulse waveform 89
unilateral ECT 60–61, 72
upper airway obstruction 43
upper respiratory tract infection 43

ventilation, during anaesthesia 46
vigabatrin 54
viloxazine 50
violent behaviour 9, 30

waiting room 37
weakness 67

young people as patients 18–21

zimeldine 50